COLOR DOPPLER FLOW IMAGING
AND OTHER ADVANCES IN DOPPLER ECHOCARDIOGRAPHY

DEVELOPMENTS IN CARDIOVASCULAR MEDICINE

Recent volumes

COLOR DOPPLER FLOW IMAGING
and other advances
in Doppler echocardiography

edited by

J. ROELANDT, MD
Thoraxcenter, Academic Hospital Dijkzigt
Erasmus University, Rotterdam, The Netherlands

1986 **MARTINUS NIJHOFF PUBLISHERS**
a member of the KLUWER ACADEMIC PUBLISHERS GROUP
DORDRECHT / BOSTON / LANCASTER
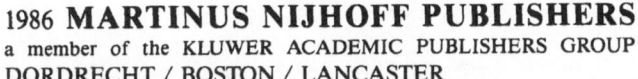

Distributors

for the United States and Canada: Kluwer Academic Publishers, P.O. Box 358, Accord Station, Hingham, MA 02018-0358, USA
for the UK and Ireland: Kluwer Academic Publishers, MTP Press Limited, Falcon House, Queen Square, Lancaster LA1 1RN, UK
for all other countries: Kluwer Academic Publishers Group, Distribution Center, P.O. Box 322, 3300 AH Dordrecht, The Netherlands

Library of Congress Cataloging in Publication Data

```
Color Doppler flow imaging and other advances in
   Doppler echocardiography.

   (Developments in cardiovascular medicine ; v.    )
   Includes index.
   1. Ultrasonic cardiography.  2. Heart--Diseases--
Diagnosis.  3. Doppler effect.  I. Roelandt, Jos.
II. Series.
RC683.5.U5C654  1986        616.1'207543        86-8647
```

ISBN-13: 978-94-010-8403-1   e-ISBN-13: 978-94-009-4283-7
DOI: 10.1007/978-94-009-4283-7

Preface

The introduction of quantitative Doppler echocardiography gave rise to explosive interest in the application of this method in clinical cardiology. However, before cardiologists could fully validate its clinical utility, they were confronted with a further development, namely color-coded Doppler flow imaging. This new technique allows a comprehensive study of the direction, velocity, uniformity and timing of intracardiac blood flow, while simultaneously revealing cardiac structures and their movement. 'Color Doppler' facilitates the diagnosis of a variety of cardiac conditions, and an overwhelming amount of information is available at any instant. Interpretation of these fascinating images requires a substantial experience and theoretical background. This monograph updates the application of color Doppler to both congenital and acquired heart disease. The work comprises 15 chapters written by authorities in the field, each of whom presents his most recent experience in the field. In addition, further advantages in the clinical use of pulsed and continuous wave Doppler in pediatric and adult cardiology are presented.

This book contains, of course, many color plates.

J. Roelandt, M.D.

Contents

VIII

III. Clinical advances in Doppler echocardiography

Contributors

S.G. van der Borden, M.D.
Thorax Center, Erasmus University Rotterdam, P.O. Box 1738, 3000 DR
Rotterdam, and Interuniversity Cardiology Institute, Utrecht, The
Netherlands
Co-authors: J. Roelandt, H. Rijsterborgh

K. Dennig, M.D.
German Heart Center, Lothstrasse 11, D-8000 München, F.R.G.
Co-author: W. Rudolph

A.B. Houston, M.D.
Department of Cardiology and University Department of Child Health,
Royal Hospital for Sick Children, Yorkhill, Glasgow 038 5J, United
Kingdom
Co-authors: I.A. Simpson, C.D. Sheldon

S. Kyo, M.D.
Department of Surgery, Saitama Medical School, 38 Moroyama-machi,
Iruma-gun, Saitama 350-04, Japan
Co-authors: S. Takamoto, E. Takanawa, M. Matsumura, Y. Yokote,
R. Omoto

R. Omoto, M.D.
Department of Surgery, Saitama Medical School, 38 Moroyama-machi,
Iruma-gun, Saitama 350-04, Japan
Co-authors: S. Kyo, S. Takamoto, M. Matsumura, Y. Yokote; from Aloka
Co., Mitaka-shi, Tokyo 181: K. Namekawa, C. Kasai, Y. Yoshikawa,
A. Koyano

C.M. Otto, M.D.
University of Washington, Division of Cardiology and Center for
Bioengineering, Seattle, WA 98195, U.S.A.
Co-authors: A.S. Pearlman, K.A. Comess, A.K. Saal, C.L. Janko,
R.R. Reamer

P. Peronneau, M.D.
Clinique Cardiologique, Unité INSERM 256, Hôpital Broussais, 96 Rue
Didot, 75674 Paris Cédex 14, France
Co-authors: B. Diebold, J.P. Guglielmi; from CGR-Ultrasonic, Meaux,
France: O. Lanusel, R. Bele, J. Souquet

J. Roelandt, M.D.
Thorax Center, Erasmus University, P.O. Box 1738, 3000 DR Rotterdam,
and Interuniversity Cardiology Institute, Utrecht, The Netherlands
Co-authors: W.B. Vletter, H. Rijsterborgh, W.J. Gussenhoven

H. Rijsterborgh, M.D.
Thorax Center, Erasmus University, P.O. Box 1738, 3000 DR Rotterdam,
and Interuniversity Cardiology Institute, Utrecht, The Netherlands
Co-author: J. Roelandt

T. Skjaerpe, M.D.
Section of Cardiology, Regional Hospital, N-7000 Trondheim, Norway

J.G. Stevenson, M.D.
Children's Hospital, Division of Cardiology, University of Washington
School of Medicine, P.O. Box C-5371, Seattle, WA 98105, U.S.A.

G.R. Sutherland, M.D.
Wessex Cardiothoracic Centre, Department of Pediatric Cardiology,
Southampton General Hospital, Shirley, Southampton SP09 4XY, United
Kingdom
Co-author: F.J. Soul

B. Wranne, M.D.
Department of Clinical Physiology, University Hospital, Regionsjuhhuset
S-581 85 Linköping, Sweden
Co-authors from Department of Biomedical Engineering, and Applied
Thermodynamics and Fluid Mechanics: P. Ask, D. Loyd

P.G. Yock, M.D.
Stanford University School of Medicine, Cardiology Division, Stanford, CA 94305, U.S.A.
Co-authors: I. Schnittger, R.L. Popp

I. Technical aspects and physical principles revisited

Structure and performances of mono- and bidimensional pulsed Doppler systems

P. Peronneau, B. Diebold, J.P. Guglielmi, O. Lanusel, R. Bele and J. Souquet

Abstract

Pulsatility of cardiac events limits the time allowed for acquiring informations. Biological tissue, ultrasonic probe and electronical circuits produce noise which is added to the signal. The theoretical accuracy of any velocity measurement can be expressed using the Woodward's relation: $s_v = k/(T_m \times R^{1/2})$, where s_v is the variance of the velocity estimation, R the signal-to-noise ratio and T_m the measurement duration. Technical problems are further complicated by the presence of wall motion producing strong low frequency Doppler signals.

In pulsed Doppler systems, transmitted bursts generate backscattered echos. Each of them is processed in order to get I and Q signals, thus defining a point. Successive bursts produce successive points, the rotation of them defining the velocity and the orientation of the target motion.

For a given depth, when a single line is studied, the number of bursts corresponding to the pulse repetition rate is used both for filtering and velocity estimation. At the opposite, when considering 2D Doppler imaging, the same number of bursts is shared between the lines required for building the image. Therefore, the number of informations available for filtering and velocity estimation is far smaller, leading to a poor accuracy.

1. Introduction

Doppler velocimeters add to the echographic analysis of structures informations about blood flows. This new dimension is of particular interest for cardiac investigations. Within the heart and the great vessels, blood motion bears informations which are useful but complex. Data obtained using either continuous wave or pulsed Doppler are too partial. An idealistic approach would access to velocimetric data in real time and in the three dimensions of the space. Any progress towards this goal is, therefore, important. Some solutions have been

4

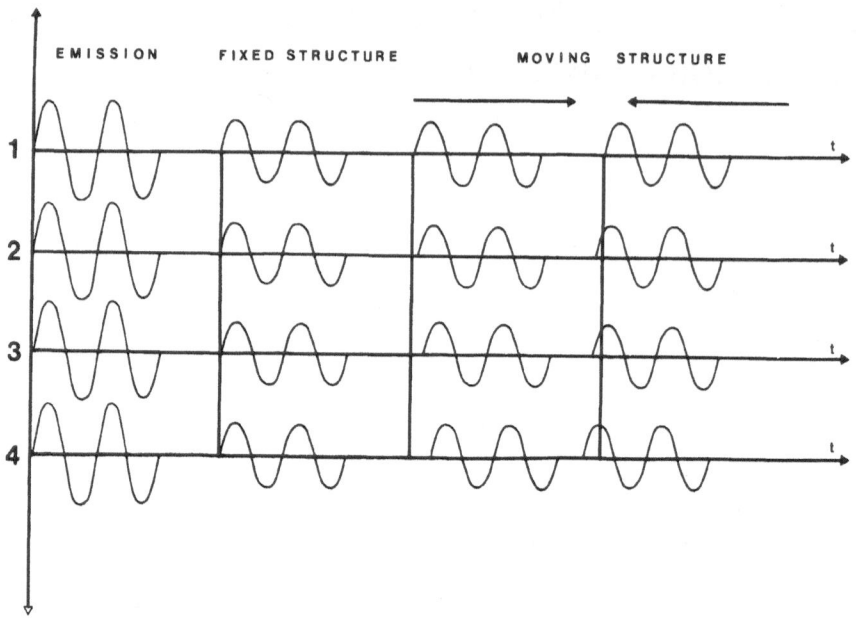

Figure 1. Schematic illustration of echos generated by four consecutive bursts. The phase of echos corresponding to a fixed structure is fixed. At the opposite, echo motion generates phase variation.

proposed, leading to simultaneous Doppler measurements in a series of points in line with the ultrasonic beam or, even, on a series of lines. When a single line is studied, a colored display allows the presentation of the time course of the measurements on the same picture in a M mode format. The same coding is used for presenting the different lines of a series in a format similar to real time 2D echo.

2. Principles

Before considering limitations, it is necessary to remind the principles involved in Doppler measurements.

The position of a given sampling site is usually assessed using the orientation of the ultrasonic beam and the distance separating the sampling site from the probe. This distance is measured by means of a pulsed emission. During each basic sequence, a brief ultrasonic burst is transmitted. Backscattered ultrasounds are analysed according to the time separating their onset from the last emission. This delay corresponds to the forth and back travel between the probe and the target.

Doppler informations are obtained by studying the modifications of backscattered bursts (Fig. 1).

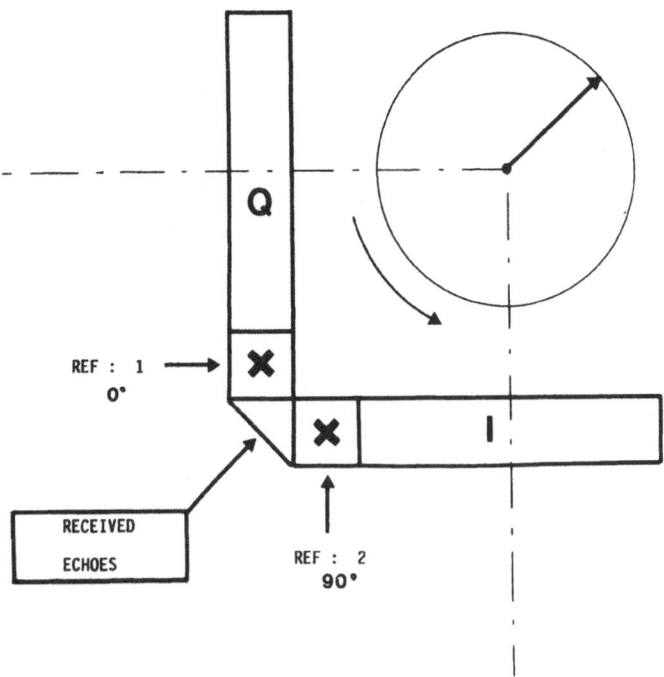

Figure 2. Illustration of echo demodulation. Received echos are multiplyed with two reference signals (REF : 1, REF : 2) in phase quadrature, producing two informations which are the abscissa and the ordinate of a point.

When considering a given immobile target, backscattered bursts are modified by the characteristics of the interface and by the attenuation within tissues. When compared to emitted bursts, their phase is different. The sequence of oscillations starts and ends with a shift. Nevertheless, successive bursts originating from the same site have the same phase and can be superposed.

When considering a mobile target, the pulse repetition rate is usually such that the shift of the target position is too low to be directly visualized using some consecutive bursts. Adversely, the phase of backscattered bursts instead of being fixed, varies. This phase shift is the basic information which can allow the reconstruction of Doppler frequencies. It is proportional to the cosine of the angle between the ultrasonic beam and the axis of the target motion.

Therefore, the analysis of echo phase is the first step for getting velocity informations using a pulsed emission. This phase analysis is generally achieved by multiplying back-scattered bursts with two different reference signals in phase quadrature. Thus, for each received burst, two brief signals are processed (Fig. 2). The two informations corresponding to each burst are the abscissa and the ordinate of a point. In case of mobile target, the successive points produced by consecutive bursts depict a rotating motion. Each point can be linked to the center by a radius, the length of which being the intensity of the Doppler signal

6

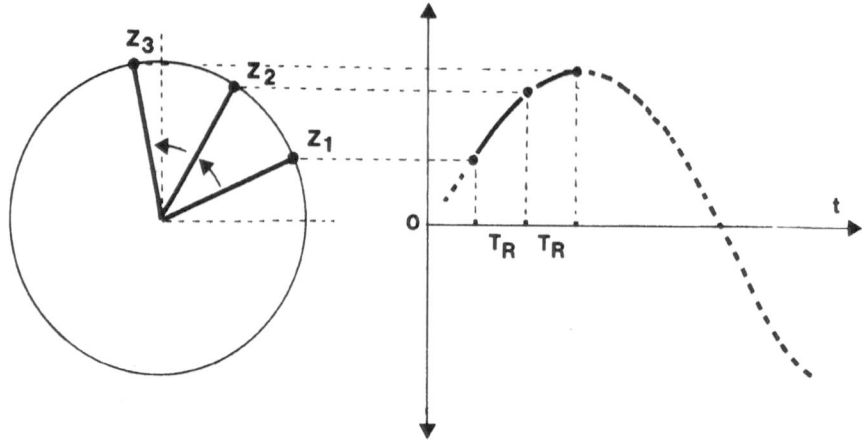

Figure 3. Illustration of the rotating motion of successive points generated by successive bursts when presented in the format of a Fresnel diagram. The time (T_r) separating consecutive points is equal to the invert of the pulse repetition rate. Doppler frequency is the projection of this motion. The angle Φ separating consecutive points is proportional to the Doppler frequency (f) and to T_r : $\Phi = 2 \cdot \pi \cdot f \cdot T_r$.

(Fig. 3). The successive radius corresponding to consecutive points define angles proportional to the velocity. The apparent orientation of the rotation indicates, in the absence of aliasing (cf. infra), the blood flow direction. The projections of this rotating motion give the Doppler frequencies, each frequency requiring a full revolution. Therefore, using the angles, velocities can be estimated without generating genuine Doppler frequency.

This accumulation of data during a given period of time together with the presence of background noise limit theoretically the accuracy of velocity measurements. As emphasized by Woodward [1], even an idealistic processor would display values with imprecisions. Any displayed value is accurate within a range which is determined by the signal-to-noise ratio (R) and the duration (T_m) of the measurement, i.e., the number of bursts accumulated for calculating the value, as follows:

$$s = K/(T_m \cdot R^{1/2})$$

where 's' is the uncertainty and K a constant. Therefore, the higher the signal-to-noise ratio and the longer the duration of a measurement, the lower the variance and the more precise the value. Adversely, with a low signal-to-noise ratio and a small amount of bursts, velocity measurements have a poor accuracy (cf. *infra*).

3. Limitations

The limitations are related to the analysed flows, the heart motion, the surrounding tissues, the ultrasonic transducer, the electronic circuitry and the algorithms used for processing the signal. Namely, it is necessary to consider the fluid mechanics, the sample volume, the aliasing, the wall motion, the signal-to-noise ratio, the time allowed for each measurement, the velocity estimators and the display protocols.

3.1 Fluid mechanics

Cardiac lesions can be described in terms of volumic flow changes, flow pattern modifications and jet development.

Volumic flow changes compensate regurgitation or are related to variations of the cardiac output. Modifications of flow pattern may be direct like in atrial septal defect or the consequence of a jet. Jets appear in almost any stenosis or regurgitation but also in shunts like ventricular septal defect or patent ductus arteriosus.

A jet is made of three regions: a central laminar cone, a secondary flow surrounding its origin and a diverging cone of turbulences progressively invading the central one. The length of the laminar cone is about four time its width. Its velocity may exceed 6 m/s. When considering a period of 10 to 20 ms, it is made of a relatively stable velocity which has the same value and orientation within the whole volume, therefore producing a narrow spectrum of Doppler frequencies. At the opposite, within turbulences, velocity varies extremely rapidly in value and orientation. The velocities measured in two nearby points are different. The corresponding Doppler spectrum is wide, the calculation of a mean velocity is very difficult.

Those phenomenon are further complicated by the physiological pulsatility which induces time variations. The Doppler signal may be considered as stable only during short periods of time. This limitating the duration of each measurement to 5 to 20 ms.

3.2 Sample volume

Physically, each Doppler measurement is performed within a volume usually named sample or measurement volume. Its width is determined by the structure of the probe and depends on the distance from the transducer and defines the lateral resolution. Its length is determined by the duration of the emitted burst, the duration of reception and the bandwidth of the equipment. Schematically, the larger the number of cycles within the emitted burst, the more accurate the measurement but the poorer the longitudinal resolution.

8

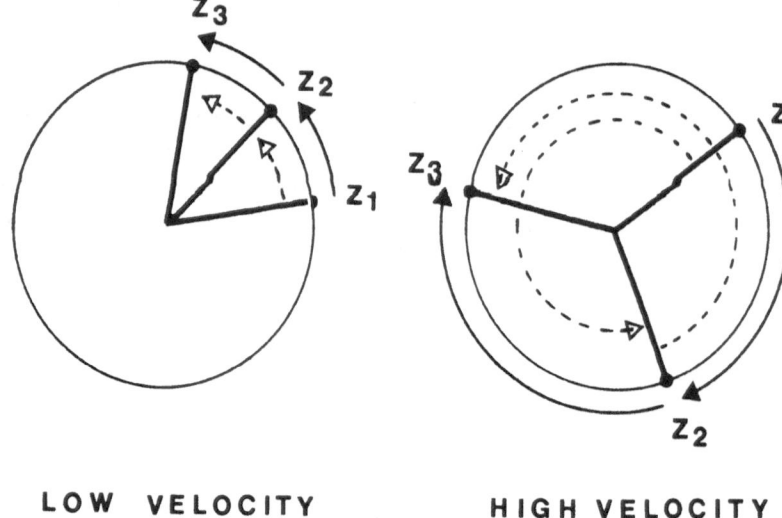

LOW VELOCITY   **HIGH VELOCITY**

Figure 4. Illustration of basic phenomenon accounting for aliasing. In case of low velocity, the rotating point describes a small angle during the time T_r separating consecutive bursts. At the opposite, in case of high velocity, the angle may exceed 180°, giving an apparent orientation of the motion (continuous line) opposed to the real (dotted line). The limit of 180° corresponds to a Doppler frequency such that $2 \cdot \pi \cdot f \cdot T_r = \pi$. Thus defining the Nyquist limit where $f = 1/(2 \cdot T_r)$.

Moving blood cells transit across the sample volume during a limited period which is inversely proportional to their velocity. This transit time may widen the Doppler spectrum. Nevertheless, this spectrum can be considered as representative of the velocity distribution provided that the sample volume is uniformly sonicated and the backscattering is assumed to be a first order phenomenon.

3.3 Aliasing

The longer the time separating two consecutive bursts, the larger the angle between the two corresponding measurements. When it is more than 180°, the apparent orientation of the velocity may be inverted and the absolute value is underestimated by, at least, 180°. This is the source of the so called 'aliasing' which may occur with any pulsed apparatus and which strongly limits their capability for measuring high velocities (Fig. 4).

3.4 Wall motion

The edges of the sample volume are not well defined. They are fuzzy. Schematically, the sample volume is made of concentric volumes, the sensitivity decreasing from the center to the periphery. This description is a major concern

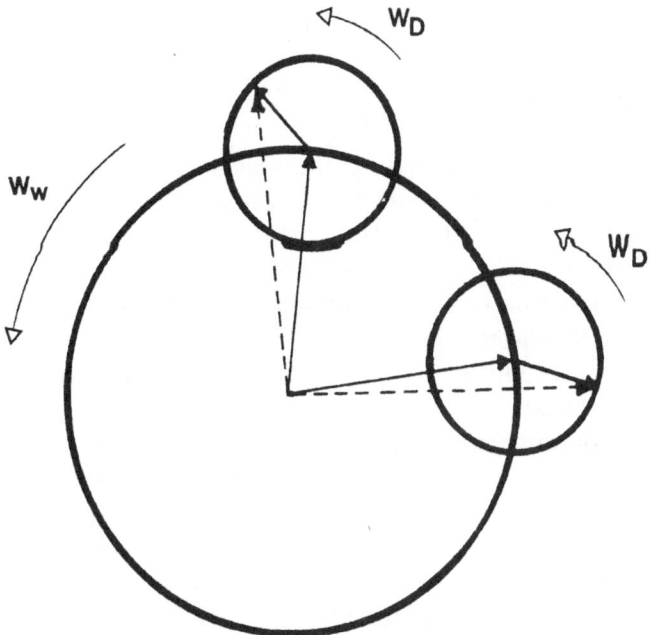

Figure 5. Fresnel diagram illustrating the influence of wall motion on two consecutive demodulated signals. Blood Doppler signal (W_D) is portrayed by small circles due to its lower energy, wall motion (W_W) is illustrated by the large central. Resulting points are obtained by the addition (dotted lines) of initial vectors (continuous lines).

for walls since their echos are far greater than those backscattered by blood cells. The energy of the Doppler signal generated by a wall, in the center of the sample volume, is 100 to 1000 times this of blood cells, i.e. 40 to 60 dB. Therefore, a moving wall may be detected even if it is apparently at distance from the sample volume. When considering successive bursts, a wall moving close to the sample volume generates successive points rotating slowly on a large circle. With the same conditions, blood motion gives rise to a smaller radius due to its lower energy but to a larger angle due to its usually higher velocity. The combination of this two components is the resulting parameter which is really processed and the modification induced by the wall motion on the velocity estimate depends on the relative size and phase of the two components (Fig. 5). Thus, for blood motion study, wall signals impose the introduction of filters that reject, as much as possible, wall components. The higher is the number of bursts considered for this purpose, the more efficient the rejection. Nevertheless, even in idealistic conditions, the rejection is limited by the fact that some wall velocities are higher than some contributive blood velocity parameters.

3.5 Signal-to-noise ratio

The received energy depends, at least, of two main factors: the emitted energy and the characteristics of ultrasound transmission within tissues.

The emitted energy is the product of the instantaneous power by the duration of the burst. This energy is limited by the heating of the transducer, the limits insuring the safety of the technic and the required resolution. The relative amount of backscattered energy increases with the emitted frequency.

Both emitted and backscattered ultrasound are attenuated while travelling within tissues. The higher the emission frequency, the more important the attenuation. Numerically, the latter is of 2 dB/MHz/cm within tissues and 0.4 dB/MHz/cm within blood.

The sources of noise are numerous. One part is produced by the analysed tissues. The probe, itself, is a source of noise, depending on its technology. In fact, a multicrystal transducer, drived using phase shifts, like in phased area imagers, introduces additional noise. This noise is further amplified through the initial amplifiers. The more sensitive the transducer, the smaller the necessary amplification and the better the signal-to-noise ratio.

When considering successive points corresponding to successive bursts, the noise introduces an additional random motion which is far from negligible in case of low signal-to-noise ratio. Therefore, the rotation of the detected points, already modified by wall motion becomes fuzzy due to the presence of noise.

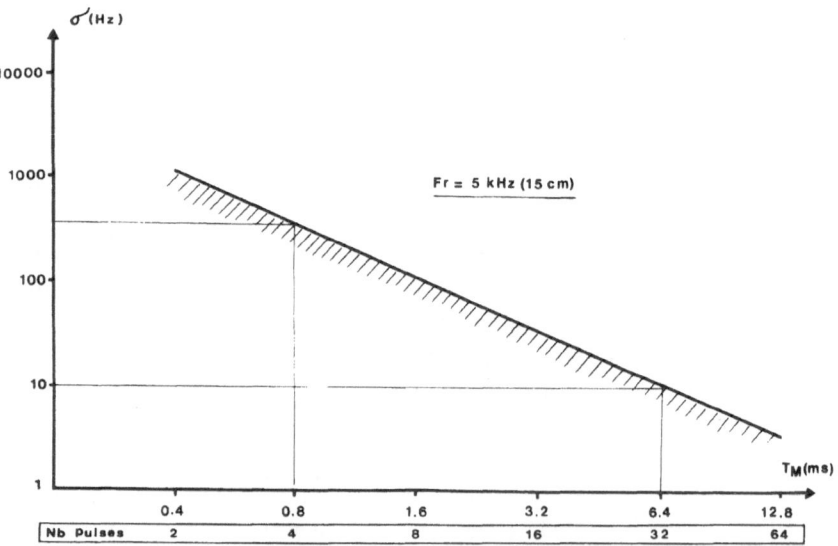

Figure 6. Theoretical relationship between the number of studied bursts and the standard error of the estimate of the mean frequency, calculated using Woodward's formula for a depth of 15 cm corresponding to a pulse repetition rate of 5 kHz and for a signal-to-noise ratio within the range usually encountered during clinical examination.

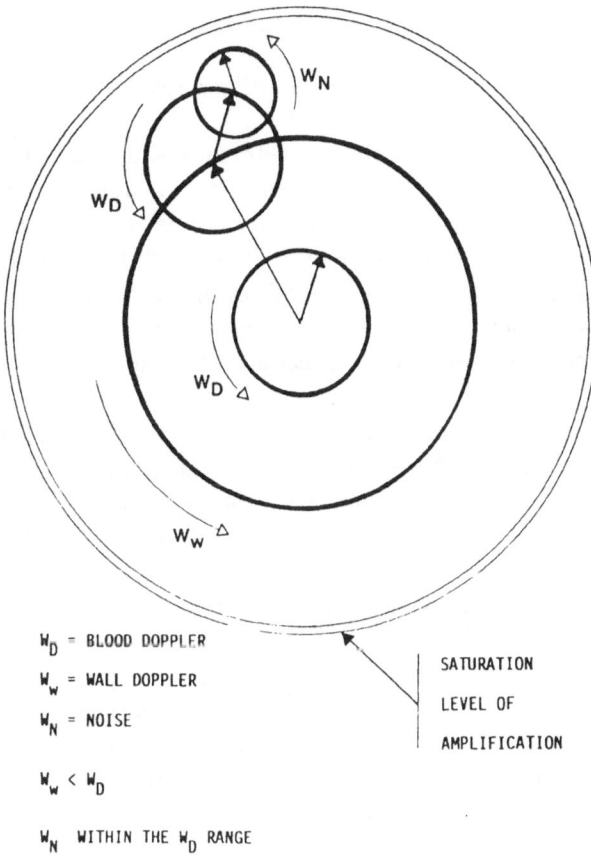

W_D = BLOOD DOPPLER

W_W = WALL DOPPLER

W_N = NOISE

SATURATION

LEVEL OF

AMPLIFICATION

$W_W < W_D$

W_N WITHIN THE W_D RANGE

Figure 7. Illustration of the sum of artifacts which is added to the studied blood Doppler signal (W_D).

3.6 Measurement time

As mentioned about principles, the duration of each measurement is a major determinant of the accuracy of velocity measurements. Its maximal value is determined by the pulsatility. Its real value depends on the used technology. When the analysis is continuously performed on the same line, like in single or multigate pulsed Doppler velocimeters, approximately 32 to 256 bursts can be processed for each measurement. At the opposite, when successive lines are very rapidly screened, the number of bursts available for each line is smaller, usually about 8. The theoretical relationship between the uncertainty of each measurement and the number of bursts involved in the measurement can be calculated, postulating a given signal-to-noise ratio. The real uncertainty being even higher (Fig. 6).

3.7 Estimators

The sequence of detected data, including artifacts related to aliasing, wall motion, noise and amplification saturation (Fig. 7), is processed using estimators.

Fast Fourier transform processors and their equivalents attempt an extraction of the different Doppler components and a display of the velocity spectrum. They need a great number of bursts. Their frequency resolution depends on the duration of individual measurements (5 to 20 ms) and their dynamic is, often, rather small when compared to the dynamic of the Doppler signal. Due to the limited duration of measurement, a velocity spectrum is only approximated by calculating the mean of many Doppler spectra, each of them being a kind of rough estimate.

Zero crossing counters require about the same duration of signal. They reduce the information by processing an instantaneous quadratic mean value and, in some cases, an evaluation of the standard deviation of the signal.

Covariance analysis [2] proposes the same data reduction but appears less sensitive to the signal-to-noise ratio. Furthermore, it may operate using a small number of bursts and has been introduced, for this reason in 2D Doppler velocimeters [3].

Beside a possible data reduction, all these estimators have their intrinsic imprecisions. These concern all the displayed values, in particular, the evaluation of the mean and, to a greater extent, the standard deviation of the signal. Indeed, the displayed variance is a combination of hemodynamic instability, signal artifacts and processor related uncertainty.

3.8 Display protocols

Data obtained in a single sample volume have three dimensions: the time, the frequency and the energy. To be presented on pictures, those data need one axis of the plane for the time, the other for the frequency and the third dimension is obtained through a grey scale or a color coding.

When considering a series of simultaneous measurements acquired along a given axis, the display should introduce a fourth dimension: the depth. Therefore, it is necessary to reduce the information. Insofar as the time is useful, frequency and energy are summarized into a single value. This reduction is, usually, achieved by calculating instantaneous mean values. Thus the influence of estimator accuracy.

In case of 2D Doppler measurement, the time course of the data can no longer be displayed on a single picture (Fig. 8).

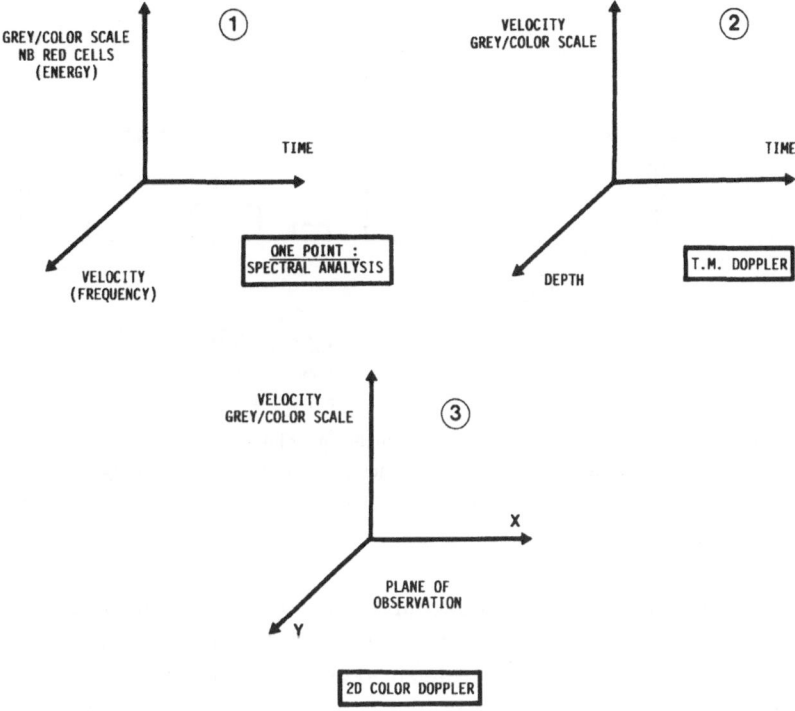

Figure 8. Schematic illustration of limitations related to display protocols.

4. Apparatus

4.1 Doppler velocimeters operating on one line

They allow a simultaneous analysis in a series of sample volumes distributed along the ultrasonic beam. Most of them have a pulsed emission according to the principle used in standard single gate velocimeters. Nevertheless, the introduction of a coded continuous emission has been proposed.

Multigate pulsed Doppler velocimeters have a general structure which can be schematically divided in three blocks: Doppler detection, wall movement filtering and blood Doppler information processing.

The Doppler detection transforms the high frequency signal produced by the transducer into informations having a lower frequency. Its general structure is about the same in all the apparatus. It is made of an amplification followed by a demodulation which is achieved by multiplying the received signal with two reference signals in phase quadrature.

The wall motion filtering is the site of the most striking differences between the apparatus and, furthermore, seems to be a key point in determining their performances. Two different principles have been developed. One is based on

14

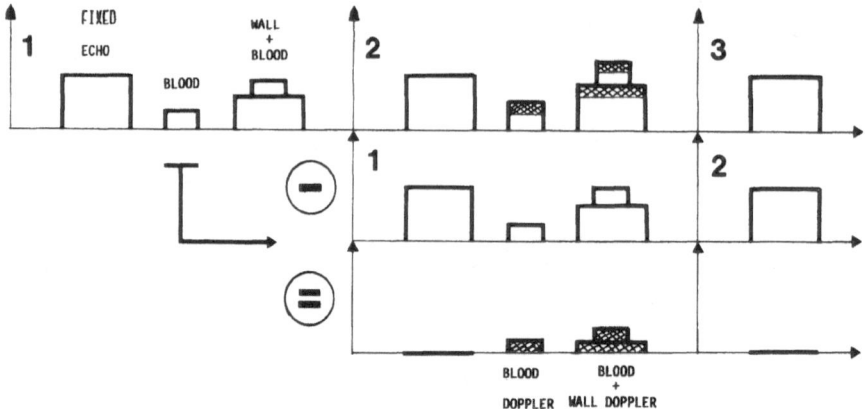

Figure 9. Principle of moving target identification. On the upper line, informations generated by three consecutive bursts are schematically displayed, dashed area corresponding to Doppler. The second line illustrates the substraction between successive data (2–1, 3–2, . . .). The lower line shows the results.

analogical filters (or their numerical equivallents) operating on the reconstituted Doppler frequencies. The other, often called M.T.I. (moving target identification), compares directly successive detected informations corresponding to successive emitted bursts.

Among the apparatus using an analogical filtering two solutions have been used: a parallel or a serial processing. The parallel structure was firstly introduced [4, 5] using, in practice, the full structure of a single gate pulsed Doppler for each sample volume. The N channels corresponding to the N gates have only two common points: the transducer and the simultaneous display of the results. Such a multiplication of circuits had induced very few industrial developments.

Recently this parallel structure has been improved by the introduction of a serial processing of filtered Doppler signals. The main advantage of this composite scheme is its unique capability to operate using filters comparable to those included in single gate pulsed Doppler velocimeters.

The full serial structure requires an analog-digital conversion of the signal immediately after demodulation [6]. I and Q signals are sampled and digitized. The limitation of the bandwidth and the filtering are sequentially achieved using numerical functions. The performance of the latter determining the performance of the apparatus.

M.T.I attempts to reject wall signals before the reconstitution of Doppler frequencies [7, 8]. The principle is to substract the values of a given point from those of the previous (Fig. 9), assuming that the higher the velocity, the larger the difference. After this procedure, the frequencies are estimated from the phase values. In some apparatus, this estimation is linear, in some others, it requires a correction. Depending on the estimator, the bandwidth is limited to one fourth of the pulse repetition rate [9] instead of the usual half. The main interest of this

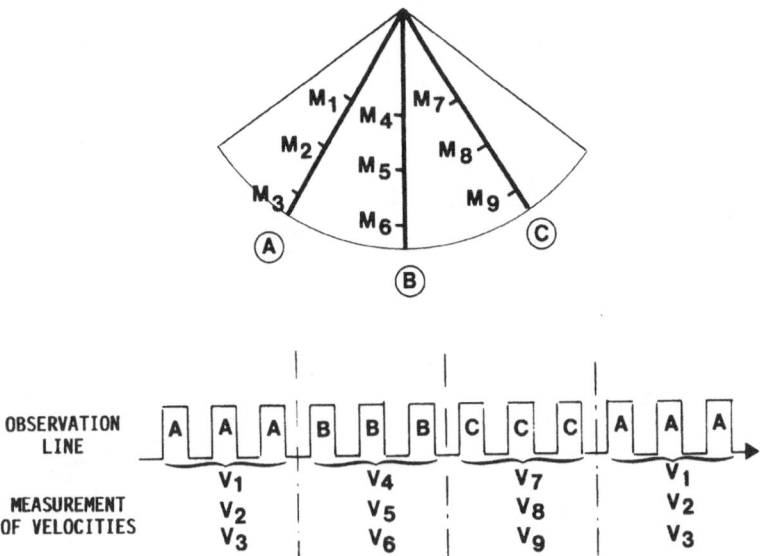

Figure 10. Principle of color flow mapping. On this scheme, the frame is made of three lines (A, B, C) with three measurement volumes (M) on each line. For building a frame, three bursts are emitted along the line A, allowing velocity estimation (V1, V2, V3) in the three measurement volumes (M1, M2, M3), then, line B and C are sequentially studied with the same protocol giving rise, respectively, to V4, V5, V6 and V7, V8, V9. The aquisition of the next frame starts at line A.

principle is its unique capability to operate using a small number of bursts. Thus, this principle has been introduced and further developed in 2D Doppler velocimeters. Its drawback is its limited effectiveness when used as a single substraction.

When using coded continuous wave emission, the phase of continuously transmitted ultrasound is coded using a pseudorandom sequence [10]. Doppler informations are obtained by correlating emitted and received signals. Those detected informations undergo a parallel processing according to their position with respect to the emitted code.

4.2 Bidimensional Doppler

The development of 2D color coded Doppler informations superimposed on 2D echo images is of great interest for cardiac studies. Moreover, this display has the particular feature of presenting data in a format similar to angiographic informations. Nevertheless, the limitations are numerous.

Each frame is obtained by sequentially studying a given number of lines exactly like echo images (Fig. 10). The values requested for producing a line are processed using a series of bursts. The time separating consecutive bursts is defined

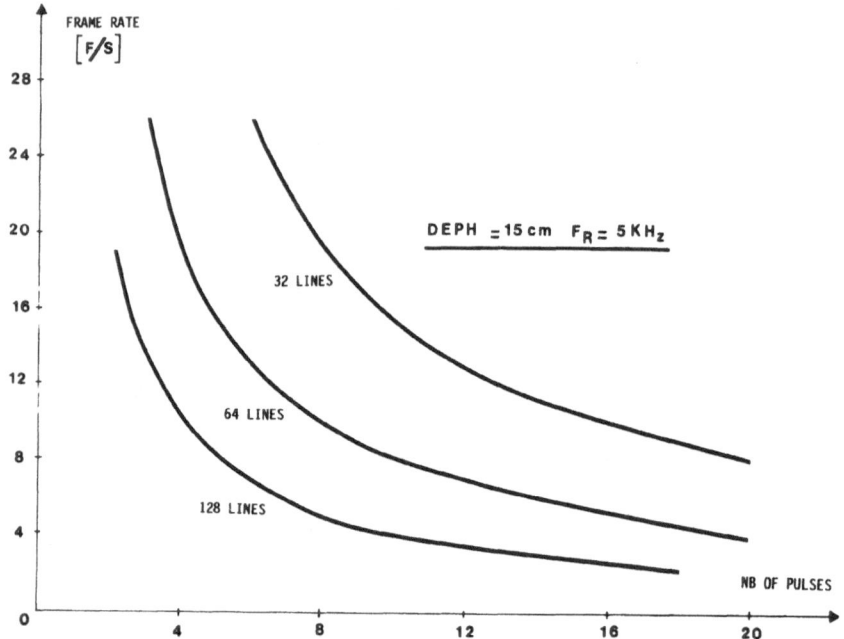

Figure 11. Calculated drawing of the hyperbolic relationship between the number of pulses per line and the frame rate for a given pulse repetition rate and different number of lines per frame.

by the pulse repetition frequency (P.R.F.) which is selected according to the analysed depth (d):

$$P.R.F. = 2 \times c/d \qquad \qquad (a)$$

where c is the velocity of ultrasound propagation in the tissues. The frame rate (F), the number of lines used for constructing each frame (L) and the number of bursts available for each line (B) are related according to the following formula:

$$P.R.F. = F \times L \times B \qquad \qquad (b)$$

defining, for a given depth and a given number of lines per frame, an hyperbolic relationship between the number bursts per line and the frame rate (Fig. 11). The combination of (a) and (b) together with the relationship between aliasing and P.R.F. illustrate the relationship between the depth and the overall quality of 2D color coded Doppler analysis. Indeed, F, L, B are the basic components of image significance in spite of possible improvement using image processing.

Due to the pulsatility of cardiac events, the interpretation of cardiac images is difficult with a frame rate of less than about 16 per heart cycle. Thus, the frame rate should be in many cases higher than 20 f/s or even 30 f/s in children. This limitating the number of lines per frame and the number of bursts per line.

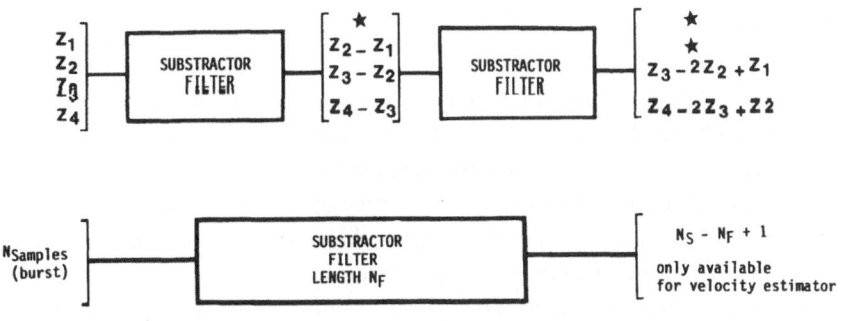

COMPROMISE BETWEEN WALL FILTERING AND VELOCITY ESTIMATION ACCURACY

Figure 12. Illustration of the compromise between filtering and velocity estimation accuracy. Each substraction improves filtering but decreases the number of data available for velocity estimation.

The limited number of lines impose a limited angle of investigation insofar high measurement accuracy is searched.

The number of bursts on each line interfers both with the efficacy of wall rejection and the accuracy of velocity estimators. As already mentioned, wall rejection is achieved using some kind of M.T.I. With a 1st order M.T.I., each detected point is substracted from the previous, N points giving rise to N-1 values. These substracted values are submitted to the same kind of operation in order to improve the filtering. Schematically, the higher the filtering efficacy, the larger the number of points devoted to this operation and the lower the number of values available for velocity estimation (Fig. 12). Adversely, the higher the number of values, the more accurate the estimation of the mean and the lower the standard error of the estimate. Therefore, a compromise is necessary in sharing the number of bursts between wall rejection and velocity estimation. As a matter of fact, the usual analog filtering corresponds to several tens substractions, this illustrating a clear theoretical difference between one line- and 2D-Doppler velocimeters.

Although some preliminary experiments have been drawn using a mechanical sector imager [3], phased array imagers seem [11] to induce fewer artefacts in spite of the above mentioned additional noise they introduce so far. This technique is the only to allow a fixed orientation of the ultrasonic beam, during the emission of the sequence of bursts along a given line, and a very rapid change of the beam orientation before the onset of the next sequence. At the opposite, the beam of a mechanical imager is continuously moving and the transit time of fixed echos generates significant Doppler signals. Furthermore, velocity estimators are less efficient when lines are not uniformly sonicated during the sequence of bursts.

Finally, the relationship between measured values and velocities is, in any case, a projection and depends on the angle between the ultrasonic beam and the blood stream lines. When considering a 2D Doppler frame, this angle varies from left to right within the frame.

18

5. Conclusion

Simultaneous echo and Doppler imaging requires, so far, a pulsed ultrasound emission which induces limitations related to the pulse repetition rate. Aliasing is present in all those techniques. When going from single to multigate systems, the basic quality of Doppler signal may remain the same but informations have to be summarized. When considering 2D Doppler, the same number of bursts is shared between a given number of lines, leading to a decrease of the accuracy of single measurements within the frame. The various systems are, therefore, complementary than substitutive and cannot substitute one another.

References

1. Woodward PM: Probability and information theory with application to radar. London: Pergamon Press, 1953.
2. Miller KS, Rochwarger MM: A covariance approach to spectral moment estimation. IEEE Trans. Inform. Theory, IT-18: 588–596, 1972.
3. Namekawa K, Kasai C, Tsukamoto M, Koyano A: Realtime bloodflow imaging utilizing autocorrelation techniques. In: Lerski RA, Morley P (eds) Ultrasound '82, pp. 203–208. Oxford: Pergamon Press, 1983.
4. Peronneau P, Bournat J-P, Bugnon A, Barbet A, Xhaard M: Theoretical and practical aspects of pulsed Doppler flowmetry: real-time application to the measure of instantaneous velocity profiles in vitro and in vivo. In: Reneman RS (ed) Cardiovascular applications of ultrasound, pp. 866–84. Amsterdam: North Holland Publishing Co., 1974.
5. McLeod FD: Multichannel pulse Doppler techniques. In: Reneman RS (ed), Cardiovascular applications of ultrasound pp. 85–107. Amsterdam: North Holland Publishing Company, 1974.
6. Hoeks AP, Reneman RS, Peronneau P: A multigate pulsed Doppler system with serial data processing. IEEE Transactions Sonics Ultrason., SU-28: 242–247, 1981.
7. Grandchamp PA: A novel pulsed directional Doppler velocimeter: the phase detection profilometer. In: Kazner E. et al. (eds) Proceedings of the Second European Congress on Ultrasonics in Medicine, pp. 123–132. Amsterdam: Excerpta Medica, 1975.
8. Brandestini M: Topoflow – A digital full range Doppler velocity meter. IEEE Transactions Sonics Ultrason., SU-25: 287–293, 1978.
9. Nowicki A, Reid JR. Dynamic ultasonic visualization of blood vessels and flows. Archives of Acoustics 7: 225–246, 1982.
10. Cathignol D, Fourcade C, Chapelon J-Y: Transcutaneous blood flow measurement using pseudo-random noise Doppler velocimeter. IEEE Transactions Biomed. Engg. 27: 30–36, 1980.
11. Yoshikawa Y, Koyano A: Performance of the system. In: Omoto R (ed) Real time two-dimensional Doppler echocardiography. Tokyo Shindan-to-Chiryo, 1984.

Estimation of transvalvular pressure drops by Doppler echocardiography: the Bernoulli equation revisited

H. Rijsterborgh and J. Roelandt

Introduction

More than three decades ago Gorlin and Gorlin [1] used the relationship between the pressure drop across a stenotic valve and the blood flow velocity which was already formulated by Bernoulli, a Dutch born mathematician, in the 18th century, for the calculation of the orifice area. In their approach they estimated the blood flow velocity at the orifice by an invasive pressure drop measurement. The application of Bernoulli's equation has received renewed interest because pressure drops across stenotic valves are now being estimated using non-invasive blood velocity measurements by Doppler echocardiography.

The Bernoulli equation relates the pressure drop across the inlet of an obstruction in a flow channel to the flow rate through it. Although this relationship is based on fundamental physical laws such as conservation of mass and energy, a number of assumptions are to be made when calculating of pressure drops and stenotic valves. These assumptions affect the accuracy of the results. It is the purpose of this chapter to review these assumptions and to critically assess their influences on the estimation of the pressure drop from Doppler velocity recordings.

Bernoulli's law

Let us consider a flow channel which includes a narrow segment as is diagrammatically depicted in Fig. 1. In this simple model steady flow is assumed and energy losses within the fluid are neglected. Since the volume flow at pressure tap I must be equal to the volume flow at tap II in the narrow segment, the velocity v_2 must be higher than the velocity v_1. The high velocity at pressure tap II represents a higher kinetic energy of the fluid elements compared to that of the fluid elements at tap I. According to the law of conservation of energy, the sum of the kinetic energy (due to velocity) and the potential energy (due to pressure) of the

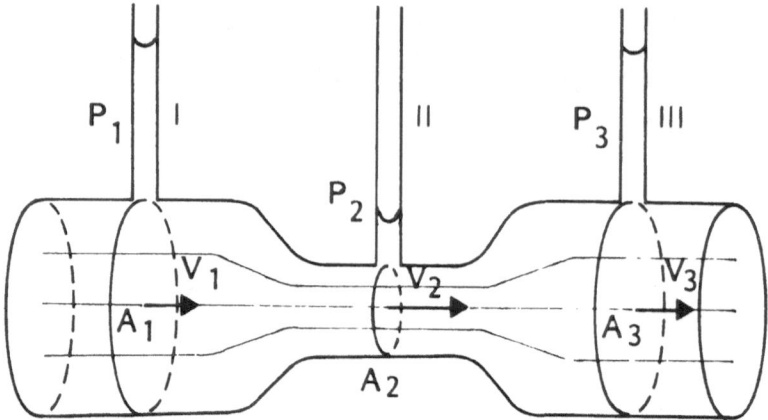

Figure 1. Model of a flow channel including a narrow segment. Without energy losses the pressure drop between tap I and tap II is fully recovered as the fluid passes from tap II to tap III and there is no pressure difference between tap I and tap III.

fluid elements must be constant everywhere in the flow channel to keep total energy constant. Therefore an increase in kinetic energy as the fluid passes from I to II can only be compensated for by a decrease in potential energy. This results in a lower pressure at tap II as compared to tap I. It is this mathematical relationship between the pressure drop and the velocities v_1 and v_2 which is described by the Bernoulli equation:

$$\Delta p = p_1 - p_2 = \frac{1}{2} \varrho \ (v_2^2 - v_1^2) \tag{1}$$

in which Δp is the pressure drop between tap I and tap II in mmHg, ϱ the fluid density in $kg \cdot m^{-3}$ and v_1 and v_2 the fluid velocities in $m \cdot s^{-1}$ at taps I and II respectively. The formal derivation of equation (1) may be found elsewhere [2].

The application of the Bernoulli equation in Doppler echocardiography to estimate pressure drops is straightforward and logic. With the Doppler instrument the blood velocity at the appropriate site of a valvular stenosis can be measured and the pressure drop can be calculated. In most patients with valvular stenosis velocity of the blood proximal to the stenosis is low relative to its velocity at the orifice. Therefore the value of v_1 may be neglected in the formula (1). The practical advantage of neglecting the proximal or upstream velocity is that the blood velocity must only be measured at the stenotic orifice. This assumption holds for most of the clinical conditions in the human heart.

By substituting the density of blood 1060 kg $\cdot$ m^{-3}) into the formula and neglecting v_1 the Bernoulli equation can be reduced to its most simple form:

$$\Delta p = 4v_2^2 \tag{2}$$

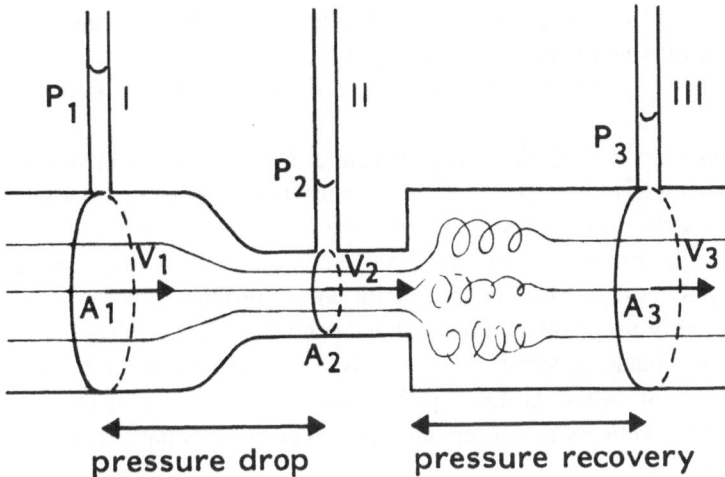

Figure 2. Model of a valvular stenosis. Between tap II and tap III most of the kinetic energy is lost due to turbulence, and the pressure is prevented from being fully recovered.

in which Δp is the pressure drop between tap I and tap II in mmHg and v_2 the blood velocity in m · s^{-1}. Note that this equation is valid when the assumptions of no energy losses and steady flow are fullfilled. It is important to realize that the Bernoulli equation only describes the relationship between velocities and pressures at the inlet of an obstruction. The pressure decreases as velocity increases due to the fact that the potential energy pressure is converted into kinetic velocity energy while total energy remains constant.

The opposite process takes place when the fluid passes from tap II to tap III and kinetic energy is again converted into potential energy. At tap III the velocity becomes lower while the pressure increases. If the flow areas at tap I and tap III are equal there will be no difference between the pressures of these respective sites. The original pressure at tap I is fully recovered and equation (2) does not describe the total pressure drop across an obstruction in a flow channel with steady flow without energy losses.

The simple model of Fig. 1, however, does not represent a genuine valvular stenosis. A valvular stenosis is marked by a sudden expansion of the cross-sectional flow area as shown by the model of Fig. 2. The abrupt outlet of the obstruction produces flow turbulence with kinetic energy losses. Full pressure recovery will thus be prevented. Thus in the application of equation (2) in order to estimate the pressure drop across a stenotic valve by Doppler echocardiography, an additional assumption must be made: pressure recovery downstream of the obstruction is zero. Only in that case the pressure at the site of the obstruction and the downstream pressure have the same value and equation (2) describes the relationship between the pressure drop across a stenotic valve and the blood velocity at the orifice of the valve only.

It appears at this stage that two assumptions contradict one another. At the inlet of the obstruction the potential energy must be converted into kinetic energy without energy losses, whereas at the outlet of the obstruction most of the kinetic energy must be lost in turbulence in order to prevent recovery. Whether both assumptions are met at the same time cannot be answered by in vivo measurements. The precise geometry of the anatomical flow channel must be known and it is impossible to obtain accurate pressure measurements in the jet area of a stenotic valve. Experience shows that a catheter cannot be held in stable position close to a stenotic orifice because of the forces produced by the jet. In vitro measurements are possible under optimal conditions and results obtained from laboratory models of stenotic aortic valves and prosthetic valves have been published [3–8]. Although these publications do not deal with Doppler echocardiographic velocity measurements, they indicate to what extend the above assumptions are valid.

Neglecting the velocity proximal to the stenosis

The omission of the velocity v_1 in equation (2) is based on the assumption that the squared value of the velocity proximal to a stenosis is very small as compared to the same value at the orifice. In the model of Fig. 2 there is a constant relationship between the velocities v_1 and v_2 which is simply dictated by the geometry of the flow channel. Since no fluid is lost the volume flow rate must be constant throughout the flow channel. In mathematical terms this means that $v_1 \cdot A_1 = v_2 \cdot A_2$. This implies that the relationship between the velocities v_1 and v_2 can be derived as being $v_1 = v_2 \cdot A_2/A_1$. The substitution of v_1 into equation (1) gives:

$$p_2 - p_1 = \tfrac{1}{2} \varrho \, v_2^2 \, (1 - (A_2/A_1)^2) \tag{3}$$

The bracketed term is determined by the ratio between the cross-sectional areas at tap I and II and independent of the velocity v_2. Note that if $A_2^2 \ll A_1^2$ the squared ratio of the cross-sectional areas can be neglected. Equation (3) is than similar to the simplified Bernoulli equation. This illustrates the identity of the assumptions $v_1^2 \ll v_2^2$ and $A_2^2 \ll A_1^2$.

It is clear from equations (1) and (3) that neglecting the velocity proximal to the obstruction results in an overestimation of the actual pressure drop. This overestimation is independent of the velocity at the site of the obstruction but determined by the ratio between the cross-sectional flow area at the obstruction and the cross-sectional flow area proximal to the obstruction.

The ratio of the cross-sectional flow areas will differ from one valve to another in the heart and from one patient to another. In addition, the ratio is not constant during the phase of flow of the cardiac cycle. In order to illustrate the importance of this cross-sectional flow area ratio in a specific patient we give the following example. Let us suppose a patient has a mild aortic stenosis and an orifice area of 1.5 cm². For sake of simplicity the left ventricle is represented by a cylindrical tube in systole with a cross-sectional area of 7 cm². The squared ratio of the cross-sectional flow areas is then 0.05. This result is an overestimation of the pressure drop by about 5% due to neglecting the velocity v_1 in the calculation. It is clear that the overestimation will decrease with decreasing orifice areas.

The most obvious solution of this problem is given by Doppler echocardiography itself. Using pulsed Doppler echocardiography the velocity in the region proximal to stenosis can be measured. Since the velocity is assumed to be low the Doppler velocity signal will not be affected by aliasing in most cases. Doppler echocardiography offers the investigator the opportunity to decide by himself whether or not to include the velocity proximal to the stenosis in the calculation of the pressure drop.

Energy losses at the inlet of the stenosis

Clark [3] formulated a theory relating the pressure difference across a stenosis to the flow through it. He described the processes that occur at the inlet region and at the area distal to the obstruction. In a laboratory model the theory was tested. Several nozzle designs were used to represent different degrees in severity of the stenosis. When energy losses at the inlet were considered the following relationship could be derived when the fluid passes from tap I to tap II in Fig. 2.

$$p_2 - p_1 = \frac{1}{2} \varrho \, v_2^2 / C_d^2 \tag{4}$$

The velocity proximal to the obstruction is assumed to be low as compared to the velocity at the site of the stenosis. The energy losses at the inlet region are represented by the nozzle coefficient C_d. The value of the nozzle coefficient varies from 1 to 0 with increasing energy losses. A nozzle coefficient which equals one corresponds to a situation without energy losses. The equations (4) and (2) are then identical.

In (3) the results are published where the nozzle coefficients of various nozzle shapes are determined. The best nozzle shape with regard to minimal energy losses reached a nozzle coefficient close to 0.9. This means that an increase in pressure drop of 19% must be taken into account due to energy losses only. Therefore, even when using water as a flowing fluid and a conical tapered inlet of the obstruction the energy losses at the inlet should not be neglected. If in the experiments the velocity at the site of the obstruction would have been measured accurately by a Doppler and used in equation (2) applied with the assumption of no energy losses, the actual pressure drop would be underestimated by 19%.

The question arises whether these results would have been different if blood had been used as a test fluid, instead of water. Blood is a mixture of fluid and small particles and its viscosity is higher as compared to water. Yoganathan et al [7] published data on pressure drops across prosthetic valves measured in a laboratory set-up. Two different test fluids were used: water and a polyol solution, which has approximately the same viscosity as blood. Their results indicate that the error of the pressure drops obtained with the polyol solution and water were similar (± 0.5 mmHg). They concluded that the viscosity of the fluid has little influence on the energy losses within the physiologic range of viscosities.

Two conclusions can be made here. Firstly, even under optimal conditions (shape of inlet), the energy losses are considerable. Secondly, the energy losses vary with the size and the shape of the obstruction in the flow channel. In clinical practice the size and the shape of the stenosis will vary from patient to patient. The extend of the underestimation of the pressure drop by Doppler echocardiography across the inlet of the stenosis remains an uncertain factor.

Pressure recovery distal to the stenosis

As already mentioned the Bernoulli equation describes the relationship between the pressure drop across the inlet of the obstruction ($p_2 - p_1$ in Fig. 2) and the velocity at the site of the obstruction. In order to calculate pressure drops across an obstruction ($p_3 - p_1$ in Fig. 2) from blood velocity measurements the assumption must be made that distal to the stenosis the pressure remains constant with distance ($p_3 - p_2 = 0$).

Both Clark [3] and Yoganathan [7] have studied the area distal to the obstruction in their respective laboratory models. In the model of aortic stenosis as well as in the prosthetic valve model considerable quantities of presure recovery were observed. In the region distal to the nozzle or prosthetic valve the pressure gradually increases. In case of the model of aortic stenosis the pressure recovery extended to 9 cm downstream of the nozzle. The results of the prosthetic valve study indicated that the region of pressure recovery extended to 15 and 27.5 cm downstream of the valve.

On the basis of the experimental measurements an expression for the total pressure recovery was derived [3]. The equation is related to the velocity at the site of the obstruction:

$$p_3 - p_2 = \varrho \, v_2^2 \left(\frac{A_2}{A_3} - \left(\frac{A_2}{A_3} \right)^2 \right) \tag{5}$$

Thus it appears that the pressure recovery is determined by the velocity at the site of the obstruction and by the ratio between the cross-sectional flow area at the obstruction and that of the flow channel distal to the obstruction.

In clinical practice the blood velocity at the orifice of a stenotic valve can be accurately measured by Doppler echocardiography. The ratio of the stenotic orifice area to the anatomical cross-sectional area distal to the valve, however, cannot be accurately measured and therefore pressure recovery is another uncertain factor in the calculation of the pressure drop across a stenotic valve.

Unsteady flow

Blood flow through the heart is basically unsteady: its velocity varies with time. As a result of the inertia of fluid c.q. blood it will take some time to accelerate or decelerate the fluid elements until the velocity dictated by equation (2) is reached. Thus, the relationship between velocity and pressure drop as described by equation (2) is lost during some phases of flow and there will be a tie delay between the velocity and the pressure drop. Unsteady flow experiments [4] have shown that the steady flow theories on pressure drop and pressure recovery are valid under unsteady flow conditions, except for a time delay between the velocity and the pressure drop.

Acceleration or deceleration of the fluid will cause a difference between the actual pressure drop and the pressure drop calculated by equation (2) which will have a delay. The instantaneous difference is described by the acceleration term which is related to the change in velocity of the fluid versus time. This corresponds to the slope of the velocity curve on the Doppler recording. A steep negative or positive slope is related to a large instantaneous difference between the actual pressure drop and the pressure drop calculated from the equation (2). In a study of patients with mitral stenosis [9] the estimate the relationship between acceleration term and the slope of the velocity recordings was calculated. Slopes up to $1 \text{m} \cdot \text{s}^{-1}$ are related to negligible errors (<0.2 mmHg) in the calculation of pressure drops.

Since the unsteady flow experiments showed good agreement with the steady flow theory on pressure drops it is obvious to calculate peak pressure drops using peak velocity measurements. At the instant of peak velocity the acceleration term is virtually zero, and the peak pressure drop will not be affected by the acceleration of the fluid. There may be a difference in timing: the moment of peak velocity will not coincide with the moment of peak pressure, but will have a small delay in time.

The consequences of a non-uniform velocity distribution

Energy losses due to friction forces at the boundary of a flow channel and friction forces within the fluid will result in a non-uniform velocity distribution across the flow area at the site of the obstruction. The introduction of energy losses and non-uniform flow profiles into the flow model will distort the relationship between the pressures and fluid velocities described by the Bernoulli equation. Due to the energy losses the actual pressure drop will be higher as compared to the pressure drop predicted by the flow rate (i.e. disregarding the energy losses). The non-uniform velocity distribution will cause dispersion of the velocities on the Doppler recording and this raises the problem which velocity measurement should be taken in the calculation of the pressure drop. In case of non-uniform velocity distribution the pressure drop is theoretically related to the spatial average of the velocities squared. Under ideal circumstances the spatial average of the velocities can be measured by a Doppler instrument. However, the square of the spatial average of the velocities is not equal to the spatial average of the velocities squared (except for plug flow). In clinical practice the blood velocity at a stenotic valve will exceed the maximal detectable velocity by a Doppler instrument.

Therefore velocities are measured by a continuous wave Doppler system assuming that the maximal velocity which is recorded originates from stenotic orifice. Due to the range ambiguity of continuous wave Doppler, no conclusions with regard to the shape of the velocity profile at the orifice area can be made from the dispersion of the velocity trace. With continuous wave Doppler only the maximal velocity can be reliably measured and a uniform velocity distribution across the orifice area is assumed by most investigators.

Discussion

A number of assumptions are made when the pressure drop across a stenotic valve is estimated by Doppler echocardiography using the simplified Bernoulli equation. Neglecting the upstream velocity in equation (2) leads to an overestimation of the pressure drop. This overestimation will decrease with smaller orifice areas of the stenotic valves. Blood velocities proximal to the stenosis can be measured with pulse Doppler and could be considered in the calculation by using equation (1).

Errors due to the unsteady flow in the heart can be reduced by avoiding pressure drop calculation during acceleration or deceleration of the blood. However, velocity slopes within a range of $\pm 1\,\text{m} \cdot \text{s}^{-1}$ are expected to produce small errors ($<0.2\,\text{mmHg}$).

Other uncertain factors influencing the accuracy of the pressure drop calculation from velocities are the energy losses at the inlet of the stenosis and the pressure recovery in the region distal to the obstruction. By combining equation (4), describing the pressure drop across the inlet including energy losses, and equation (5), which describes the pressure recovery, a formal expression regarding the actual pressure drop across a stenotic valve can be derived:

$$\Delta p = p_1 - p_3 = \tfrac{1}{2}\,\varrho\,v_2^2 \left[\frac{1}{c_d^2} - 2\,\frac{A_2}{A_3} + 2\left(\frac{A_2}{A_3}\right)^2 \right] \tag{6}$$

The subscripts refer to Fig. 2. The square bracketed term is independent of both the flow rate and velocity at the site of the obstruction and is assumed to equal one in the simplified Bernoulli equation. The net result is that the underestimation caused by neglecting the energy losses is partly compensated by the overestimation due to the pressure recovery. This may be illustrated by the following examples.

Mild aortic stenosis with an orifice area of $1.2 \, cm^2$. We assume a nozzle coefficient of 0.9 and a cross-sectional flow area of $4.9 \, cm^2$ in the aorta. The term between square brackets in equation (6) is 0.86. Thus the simplified Bernoulli equation will overestimate the actual pressure drop across the stenotic valve by 16%. Severe aortic stenosis with an orifice area of $0.5 \, cm^2$. We assume the same values of the nozzle coefficient and cross-sectional flow area of the aorta. The term in equation (6) is now 1.05. This results in an underestimation by 5% by the simplified Bernoulli equation.

Recently the results of *in vitro* studies have been published where the relationship between pressure difference and fluid velocity was analyzed [5]. The velocities at the site of the obstruction were measured with a Doppler instrument and the results of the calculation using the simplified Bernoulli equation compared with actual pressure measurements. The tests included different flow rates, different nozzle diameters and a range of fluid viscosities. It was found that the actual pressure was underestimated by the Doppler method by 4% on the average. The individual differences of the paired measurements, however, had a range of $\pm 12\%$ (two standard deviations). This indicates that in *in vitro* experiments several factors complicate the pressure drop measurements and that the application of a simplified Bernoulli equation leads to errors.

In clinical practice the estimation of the pressure drop across a stenotic valve by Doppler echocardiography and using the Bernoulli equation suffers from variability introduced by unknown factors, which tend to compensate one another.

Firstly, the energy losses at the inlet of the stenotic valve cannot be quantified in the individual patient as it is dependent upon the actual geometry of the inlet region and the shape of the valve. Secondly, the non-uniform velocity distribution will tend to overestimate the calculated pressure drop, since the measured velocity will be higher as compared to the theoretical velocity assuming a uniform distribution. Thirdly, the pressure recovery in the regio downstream of the valve cannot be measured non-invasively and depends mainly on the value of the cross-sectional flow area of the valve.

It should be realized that when pressure drops measured by catheter are compared with pressure drops estimated by Doppler echocardiography, additional variability is introduced by the pressure recovery. To obtain a good pressure recording by catheter will be positioned somewhere in the region of pressure recovery, outside the turbulent area at a variable distance from the stenotic valve. No standardization is possible and in the studies no information is available where exactly the catheter tip was positioned. It is therefore unknown which part of the pressure recovery may extend well beyond the turbulent region.

Theoretically, the most accurate estimate of the severity of a stenosis is represented by the velocity in the stenotic orifice. Thus, we may think in the future of using velocities rather than pressure drops for estimating severity and calculating the orifice area.

References

1. Gorlin R, Gorlin SG: Hydraulic formula for calculation of the area of the stenotic mitral valve, other cardiac valves, and central circulatory shunts. I. Am Heart J 41 (1): 1–22, 1951.
2. Klip W: Theoretical foundations of medical physics vol. II: an introduction into medical physics pp. 776–780. University of Alabama press, 1969.
3. Clark C: The fluid mechanics of aortic stenosis. I. Theory and steady flow experiments. J Biomechanics 9: 521–528, 1976.
4. Clark C: The fluid mechanics of aortic stenosis. II. Unsteady flow experiments. J Biomechanics 9: 567–573, 1976.
5. Holen J, Waag RC, Gramiak R, Violanti M, Roe SA: Doppler ultrasound in orifice flow. In vitro studies of the relationship between pressure difference and fluid velocity. Ultrasound in Med & Biol 11 (2): 261–266, 1985.
6. Wong M, Vijayaraghhavan G, Bae JH, Shah PM: Study of the pressure-velocity relation across stenotic orifices. Am J Cardiol 56: 465–469, 1985.
7. Yoganathan AP, Corcoran WH, Harrison ECV: Pressure drops across prosthetic aortic heart valves under steady and pulsatile flow – in vitro measurements. J Biomechanics 12: 153–164, 1979.
8. Bruss K-H, Reul H, van Gilse J, Knott E: Pressure drop and velocity fields at four mechanical heart valve prostheses: Björk-Shiley standard, Björk-Shiley concave-convex, Hall-Kaster and St. Jude medical. Life Support Systems 1: 3–22, 1983.
9. Hatle L, Brubakk A, Tromsdal A, Angelsen B: Non-invasive assessment of pressure drop in mitral stenosis by Doppler ultrasound. Br Heart J 40: 131–140, 1978.

Factors influencing fluid velocity measurements in valvular regurgitation

Bengt Wranne, Per Ask and Dan Loyd

Summary

Viscous velocity loss becomes important only at very small holes where the volume of regurgitation is negligible.

Contraction of the jet gives a lower volume flow than expected from the equation of continuity, but has only a negligible influence on the velocity in the core flow of the regurgitant jet.

Inherent properties of the spectral analysis of the Doppler signal, in combination with a small core flow volume will create difficulties in distinguishing high regurgitant velocities from background noise.

Introduction

It is a common clinical finding that, when using the continuous ultrasound Doppler, the velocity of the regurgitant jet in mitral and aortic regurgitation is lower than that expected from the approximate Bernoulli relationship

$$v \approx \frac{\sqrt{\Delta p}}{2} \qquad (1)$$

where Δp (mmHg) is the pressure difference across the valve and v the maximal velocity of the regurgitant jet.

Factors that might explain the measured lowered velocity are measurement geometry, the hydraulic conditions at the leaking hole and properties of the Doppler instrument. The aims of the present paper are:

1. to clarify the theory of these hydraulic conditions;
2. to perform a model experiment to relate pressure and flow through holes with various diameters;
3. discuss reasons for the observed velocity loss;

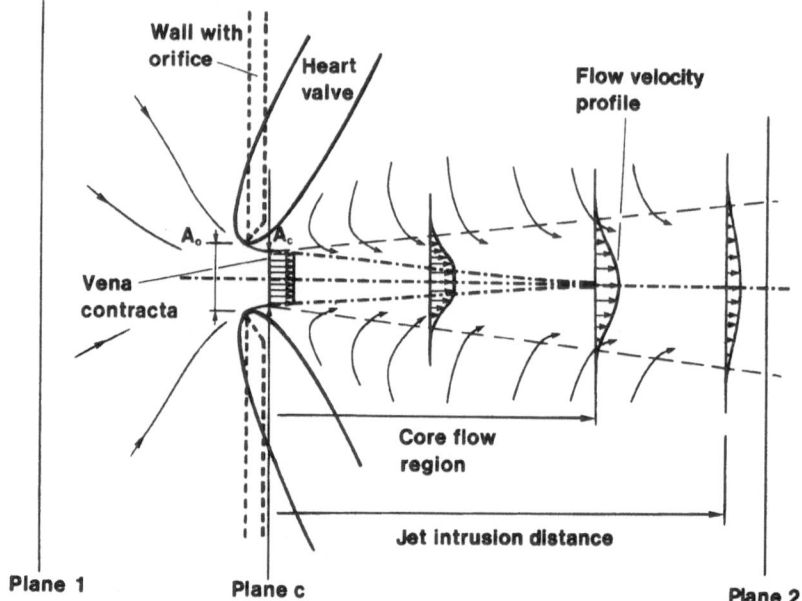

Figure 1. The regurgitant flow through a heart valve with velocity profiles and streamlines of the regurgitant jet. In the core flow region the flow velocity is equal to that at the vena contracta. Distance of jet intrusion is the distance from the orifice to a point where the velocity has decreased to a value v_x. The sharp-edged orfice model is shown together with a realistic heart valve hole. A_o is the area of the orfice and A_c the area of the vena contracta.

4. discuss possibilities and difficulties in quantifying leakage from the information contained in the Doppler signal.

Theory

We assume, as a first approximation, that a leaking heart valve can be modelled as a sharp-edged circular or slot type orfice in a plane rigid wall. The driving pressure difference over the leaking valve may vary from 3 kPa for tricuspid or pulmonary regurgitation to 25 kPa at mitral regurgitation. The diameter of the circular hole and the width of the slot orfice are both assumed to be larger than 2 mm for the regurgitant flow to be of clinical significance. For these restrictions the flow can be found to be turbulent [1].

The regurgitant flow through a leaking valve can be described as in Fig. 1. At the entrance of the orfice the flow contracts. This contraction continues and approximately half a diameter (slotwidth) downstream the orifice the area of the jet flow reaches a minimum, the so called vena contracta. The ratio between the jet area at the vena contracta, A_c, and the area of the orfice, A_o, is called the contraction coefficient, C_c [2]. That is

$$C_c = \frac{A_c}{A_o} \qquad (2)$$

In the core flow region, the length of which is normally in the order of 4–8 diameters (slot-widths), the flow velocity is equal to that at the vena contracta [3]. The total length of jet intrusion, x, defined as the distance from the orifice to which the velocity has decreased to a certain velocity, v_x is given by

$$x = k_1 \frac{\bar{v}_o \cdot d}{v_x} - k_2 \qquad (3)$$

where k_1 and k_2 are constants, $\bar{v}_o$ the average velocity at the hole and d the diameter of the hole [4, 5].

By applying the Bernoulli equation to planes 1 and c in Fig. 1, and by neglecting the flow velocity at plane 1, we get

$$v_c = \sqrt{\frac{2}{\varrho} (p_1 - p_2)} \qquad (4)$$

where v_c is the flow velocity at the vena contracta, ϱ the density of blood, p_1 the pressure at plane 1 and p_2 the pressure at plane 2. The latter pressure can be shown to be approximately equal to that at the vena contracta.

Even if equation (4) was calculated for frictionless flow, effects of viscous friction can be taken into account by using a velocity coefficient, C_v [2]:

$$C_v = \frac{v_f}{v_{fl}} \qquad (5)$$

where v_f is the actual velocity and v_{fl} the velocity corresponding to the frictionless case. For the orifice model, C_v is close to one for realistic orifice sizes and pressure differences.

From the continuity equation and equations (2) and (5) we get

$$\dot{Q} = C_v \cdot C_c \cdot A_o \cdot v_c \qquad (6)$$

where $\dot{Q}$ is the regurgitation flow.

By defining a discharge coefficient, C_d, as

$$c_d = C_v \cdot C_c \qquad (7)$$

this can be rewritten as

$$\dot{Q} = C_d \cdot A_o \cdot v_c \qquad (8)$$

Since in the described case the velocity coefficient is close to one the value of the discharge coefficient varies mainly with the degree of contraction of the flow. For the sharp-edged orifice with the diameter (slot-width) and driving pressure in the ranges described above, the discharge coefficient has empirically been found to be 0.61 [2].

If the valve hole has a considerable length in relation to its diameter (width), the model described above might not be fully applicable. If we, however, assume the hole to be circular and tube-shaped with sharp-edged entrance the discharge coefficient can be written as [2]

$$C_d = \frac{1}{\sqrt{1.5 + 13.7 \sqrt{\dfrac{l}{d \cdot Re}}}} \quad \text{for } \frac{d \cdot Re}{l} > 50 \tag{9}$$

where l is the length of the hole, d the diameter and Re the Reynolds number [6]. It can be calculated that viscous losses become important first at very small orifices where the regurgitant volume is negligible. From equation (9) one can see that viscous losses are not very sensitive to changes in length of the hole.

For the short, tube-shaped hole with sharp-edged entrance and a length/ diameter ratio larger than 2, the flow contracts at the inlet of the tube and after a vena contracta is reached inside the hole, the flow then diverges and follows the cylindrical outlet of the hole. For a length/diameter ratio below 0.5 the flow sitution is identical to that in the sharp-edged orifice. For a length/diameter ratio in the range of 0.5–2 several flow situations may occur. The flow may either behave like that of a sharpe-edged orifice or like that of a tube-shaped hole with a length/diameter ratio >2. In a third case the flow may contract inside the hole but at the outlet, the resulting jet may adhere asymmetrically to the inner surface of the outlet. This place can change e.g. to upstream external forces and the direction of the jet may therefore be unstable.

The discharge coefficient changes with the shape of the inlet mainly due to a changing contraction coefficient. For a hole with a conical inlet (cone angel equal to 50°) the contraction is less and the discharge coefficient is given by

$$C_d = \frac{1}{\sqrt{1.09 + 0.088 \dfrac{l}{d} + \dfrac{0.32}{Re^{0.25}} \cdot \dfrac{l}{d}}} \tag{10}$$

As seen from the presented discharge coefficients for orifices in rigid walls, the volume flow can be expected to be lower than the flow calculated just by using the velocity from Bernoulli's equation and the hole area. The main reason for this is contraction of the flow and not velocity losses due to friction. The velocity at the core flow region is close to that expected from the Bernoulli equation for flow situations where the regurgitation is clinically significant.

A more detailed presentation of this theory is given elsewhere [1].

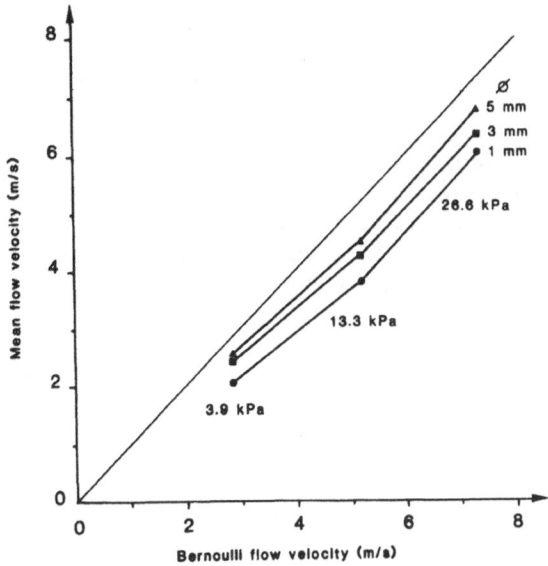

Figure 2. Mean flow velocity, obtained as measured volume flow divided by hole area as a function of the Bernoulli velocity calculated from the pressure differences. The hole diameters are 1, 2 and 3 mm. The driving pressure differences are 3.9, 13.3 and 26.6 kPa.

Model experiment

The volume flow for various hole diameters and driving pressures was studied in a model experiment where a water tank and adaptors with various hole diameters were used in a similar way as that described earlier [5]. The driving pressure was varied by varying the height of the tank relative the height of the adaptor hole. The temperature of the water was 22° C. The adaptors had hole diameters of 1.0, 2.0 and 5.0 mm and the length of the hole was 10 mm. The inlet of the hole had a conical shape with a cone angel of 115°.

The volume flow for driving pressures of 3.9, 13.3 and 26.6 kPa was measured using a measuring glass and a stop watch. The average flow velocity was calculated by dividing the measured flow with the area of the hole.

Experimental results

In Fig. 2, the mean flow velocity obtained from the measured volume flow divided by the hole area is shown as a function of the velocity obtained from the Bernoulli equation. For all hole diameters and driving pressures the measured mean flow is lower than that calculated from the Bernoulli relation. This is, according to the theory, for the 3 and 5 mm orifices due mainly to contraction of

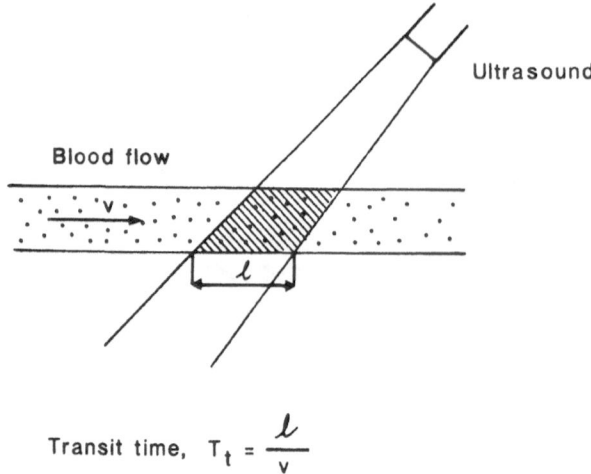

Figure 3. Ultrasound Doppler measurement of blood flow velocity. v is the velocity of the blood and l the transit length of the blood cells, i.e. the scatterers, in the ultrasound beam.

the flow, while friction becomes important at the 1 mm orifice. The maximal flow velocity of the jet can be expected to be close to the theoretical one except for the holes with the smallest diameters.

Limitations of the ultrasound Doppler technique

The limitations of the pulsed ultrasound Doppler technique for measuring high velocities and the influence of incorrect alignment of the Doppler beam with the blood flow is nowadays well known and will not be discussed here. When using the continuous Doppler technique the measurement of velocity of blood flow can in a simplified situation be described as in Fig. 3. The blood flow has a certain transit length, l, at which a blood cell is exposed to the ultrasound beam and can generate back-scattered Doppler shifted ultrasound. If the blood flow velocity is equal to v, the transit time T_t, [7] of the blood cells is given by

$$T_t = \frac{l}{v} \tag{11}$$

If one wishes to measure the maximal velocity in the case of regurgitation, the transit length will be the length of the core flow region.

The Doppler signal for a low and a high velocity flow is shown in the upper panel of Fig. 4. The high velocity flow corresponds to a higher Doppler frequency but a shorter transit time compared to the low velocity case. The number of periods of the two Doppler signals, however, are the same.

A

Doppler signals

low flow velocity

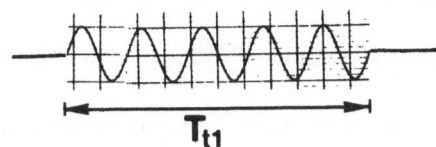

high flow velocity

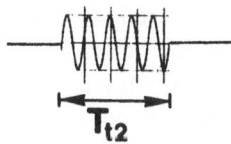

B

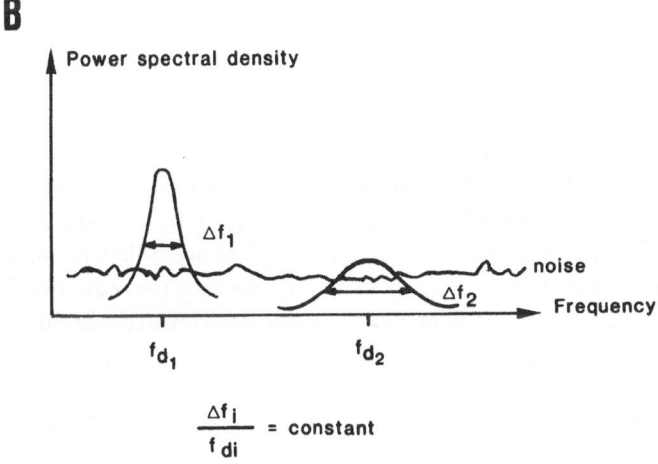

$$\frac{\Delta f_i}{f_{di}} = \text{constant}$$

Figure 4. Upper panel: Ultrasound Doppler signals for low and high velocity flow. T_{t1} and T_{t2} are the respective transit times. Lower panel: The power spectrum of the low velocity flow, Doppler frequency f_{d1}, and the high velocity flow, Doppler frequency f_{d2}. The corresponding spectral widths are Δf_1 and $\Delta f_2 \cdot \Delta f_i / f_{di}$ is independent of frequency. The noise spectrum has approximately a constant amplitude.

The two Doppler signals are samples of sine signals, the frequency spectra of which are shown in the bottom part of Fig. 4. The relative spectral widths of the two spectra are the same since the number of sine periods are equal, i.e.

$$\frac{\Delta f_i}{f_{di}} = \text{constant} \tag{12}$$

where Δf_i is the spectral width of signal i and f_{di} is the Doppler frequency of that signal.

The power spectral density of the measurement noise is approximately independent of the frequency. The quotient between the maximal power spectral density of the Doppler signal and the spectral density of the noise therefore decreases with increasing Doppler frequency. This fact makes it difficult to resolve high frequency components, corresponding to high blood flow velocities, from the noise spectrum.

The total power of a Doppler signal, for a certain velocity, is also related to the number of scatterers in a volume having that velocity. As stated in the theory section the maximal flow exists only in the core flow region, the volume of which is quite small. It might therefore be a problem to distinguish the signal eminating from this volume from the noise, especially at high flow velocities in small holes, since in this case the effects due to the limited volume are combined with the broadening of the frequency spectrum described above.

Discussion

The ultimate goal when using Doppler technique for the assessment of valve regurgitation must be the measurement of regurgitation volume. In a recent paper [5], we have shown that the distance of jet intrusion must be used with caution for this purpose since the jet intrusion distance is dependent on both the pressure difference over the valve and on the hole area (see equation 3) [4, 5]. In the same paper we also, for an idealized model, derived an equation for measurement of volume of regurgitation, V_r,

$$V_r = \frac{\Pi}{4} \frac{(v_x)^2}{k_1^2} (k_2 + x)^2 \frac{T_r}{\bar{v}_0} \tag{13}$$

where k_1 and k_2 are constants, the distance x corresponds to the distance from the valve to a point where the flow velocity is reduced to a certain value v_x; $\bar{v}_0$ is the mean velocity in the orifice and T_r the regurgitation time. Besides the constants k_1 and k_2, the right hand side of equation (13) contains only variables that, at least in the idealized situation, can be measured with ultrasound Doppler.

The potential advantage of this approach is that the diameter of the hole has been eliminated and the volume of regurgitation can be determined if $\bar{v}_o$ and x are determined, which may be done with Doppler technique. Also, the measurement technique avoids the problem with contraction outlined above in the theory section.

As the velocity through the orifice is one of the determinants in this equation it is of interest to clarify factors which have influence on this term. We have here shown viscous velocity losses become important first at very small holes with negligible regurgitation. Even so, this does not preclude the use of v_o in this respect as long as it is correctly measured. One must, however, remember that the equation is derived for an idealized model and it has yet to be proven if it, with approximations, can be used in the clinical situation.

One further matter of concern is the problem of measuring high flow velocities correctly. The importance of having the Doppler beam parallel to the regurgitant jet and the aliasing problem of the pulsed Doppler technique in this respect are by now well known [7]. As pointed out above, there are, however, problems in registering high velocities also with the continuous Doppler technique in situations where the diameter of the hole is small and consequently also the volume of the core flow region is small. This must be considered if one attempts to use equation (13) clinically.

Acknowledgement

Supported by the Swedish Medical Research Council grant 07158, the Swedish National Association against Heart and Chest Diseases and the County Council, County of Östergötland, Sweden.

References

1. Ask P, Loyd D, Wranne B: Regurgitant flow through heart valves. A hydraulic model applicable to ultrasound Doppler measurements. Medical Biological Engineering and Competing, 1986: in press.
2. Merrit HE: Hydraulic control systems; pp. 39–48. New York: John Wiley & Sons, 1967.
3. Eck B: Technische Strömungslehre, pp. 120–23. Berlin: Springer-Verlag, 1978.
4. Hinze JO: Turbulence, pp. 404–09. New York: MacGraw-Hill, 1959.
5. Wranne B, Ask P, Loyd D: Quantification of heart valve regurgitation. A critical analysis from a theoretical and experimental point of view. Clin Physiol 5: 81–8, 1985.
6. Massey BS: Mechanics of fluids, pp. 124–221. London: Van Nostrand Reinhold, 1979.
7. Hatle L, Angelsen B: Doppler ultrasound in cardiology. Physical principles and clinical applications, pp. 32–73. Philadelphia: Lea & Febiger, 1985.

Computer-aided analysis of Doppler echocardiograms

S.G. van der Borden, J.Roelandt and H. Rijsterborgh

Summary

Measurement from Doppler echocardiograms and calculation of clinically relevant parameters are most commonly performed manually. The procedure is time consuming and introduces measurement errors. Furthermore documentation of the results remains difficult when they have to be used for a clinical patient record or for research. Computer-aided analysis of Doppler echocardiograms helps to improve accuracy, and information on the variability of a specific measurement can be calculated. Uniform reports can be generated for clinical record keeping and be send to a main database system. We describe a computer-aided analysis configuration for Doppler echocardiograms using a personal computer which is linked to a digitizing tablet for input and a printer for report generation. There is an additional option of sending and retrieving data from the hospitals main database system. The system, analysis procedure and error sources in the different phases of the analysis procedure are discussed.

1. Introduction

Doppler frequency shifts or velocities sampled from selected areas within the heart show a large variability due to methodological and physological factors. This leads to a large random error whenever these Doppler velocities are used to calculate pressure drops by applying the simplified Bernoulli equation. Valve orifice area calculation when derived from pressure half time values is subject to a large measurement variability. Similarly, mean temporal velocities have both a large variability and measurement error. The predominant error in measuring the above parameters is assumed to be random and therefore it is necessary to average the data of several cardiac cycles. Indeed, the random error is reduced by the square root of the number of beats averaged. This means that when the data of nine consecutive beats are averaged the random error is reduced by a factor

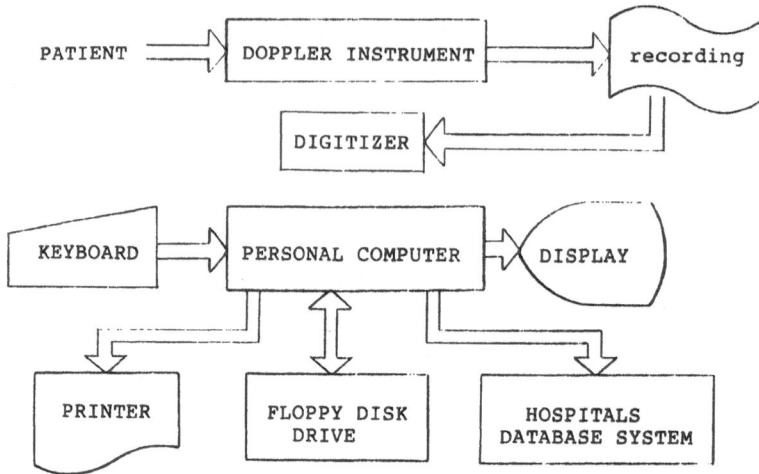

Figure 1. System blockdiagram.

three. We therefore have developed a computer aided analysis program using a digitizing tablet and an Olivetti M24 personal computer.

2. Methods

2.1 Doppler echocardiograms

Pulsed or continuous wave Doppler echocardiograms are most commonly recorded with a stripchart recorder at a paperspeed of 50 or $100 \, \text{mm} \cdot \text{s}^{-1}$. The ultrasonic frequency used may change from one system to another but for adult examination is typically 2.5 MHz. In the pulsed mode, the pulse repetition frequency may vary from 4 to 12 kHZ, allowing a maximal velocity to be measured up to $0.65 \, \text{m} \cdot \text{s}^{-1}$ at a depth of 16 cm from the transducer and up to $1.94 \, \text{m} \cdot \text{s}^{-1}$ at a depth of 3.8 cm. In the continuous mode, velocities as high as $7.75 \, \text{m} \cdot \text{s}^{-1}$ up to a depth of 16 cm from the transducer can be measured. Together with the Doppler trace calibration markers and the electrocardiogram are recorded.

2.2 System configuration (Hardware)

The analysis system consists of a personal computer (Olivetti M24), forming the core of the system, with two floppy disks for program and data storage, a digitizer (Summagraphics MM961), connected to the personal computer via a serial interface and on which the Doppler velocity contours are digitized. A printer is connected via a parallel interface for report output. A block diagram of the system is shown in Fig. 1.

2.3 System output description

Depending on the type of Doppler trace different parameters can be derived. For the mitral and tricuspid valve they are summarized in Table 1 and for the aortic and pulmonic valve in Table 2. Using the simplified Bernoulli equation the pressure drop is calculated for velocities above $1\,m \cdot s^{-1}$ because it is assumed that $v_2 \gg v_1$, whereas v_2 represents the value of the jet velocity and v_1 the velocity proximal to the stenosis [1]. Independent from the type of Doppler trace time reference parameters are calculated (Table 3). The mean values from several consecutive cardiac cycles are calculated together with their standard deviation, to give a measure of the variability.

The system is programmed in GWBASIC, PASCAL and partly in assembly language. System operation occurs interactively via dialogue.

3. Analysis procedure and definitions

Computer processing of Doppler echocardiograms requires transformation into digital form. A block diagram of the system for recording and digitization is shown in Figure 1. A semi-automatic approach is used to enter the time velocity recording into the computer. We have not chosen a fully automated system

Table 1. Derived parameter for mitral and tricuspid valve.

Physical quantity		Units	Derived from
Early diastolic velocity	EADV	$m \cdot s^{-1}$	Manual ref. point
Early diastolic gradient	EADG	mmHg	EADV
Mean diastolic velocity	MDV	$m \cdot s^{-1}$	Velocity-time integral
Mean diastolic gradient	MDG	mmHg	Pressure-time integral
End diastolic velocity	EDV	$m \cdot s^{-1}$	Manual ref. point
End diastolic gradient	EDG	mmHg	EDV
Peak systolic velocity	PSV	$m \cdot s^{-1}$	Manual ref. point
Peak systolic gradient	PSG	mmHg	PSV
Mean systolic velocity	MSV	$m \cdot s^{-1}$	Velocity-time integral
Mean systolic gradient	MSG	mmHG	Pressure-time integral
Systolic ejection period	SEP	s^{-3}	Manual ref. point
Diastolic filling period	DFP	s^{-3}	Manual ref. point
Pressure halftime	PHT	s^{-3}	EADG
Orifice area	OA	cm^2	PHT

42

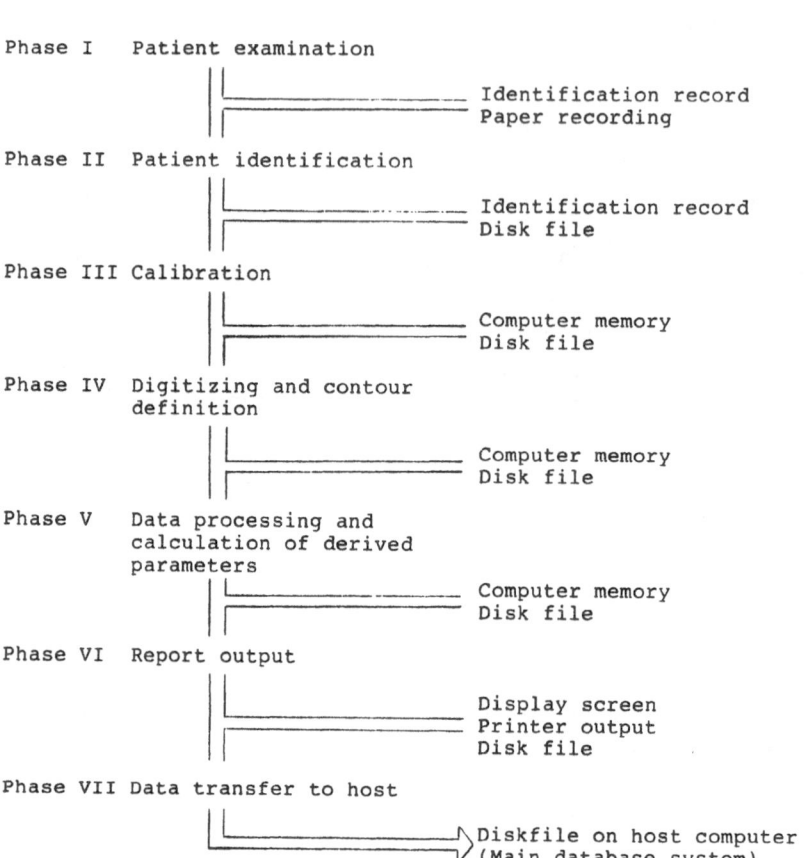

	Procedure	Output/Storage medium
Phase I	Patient examination	Identification record Paper recording
Phase II	Patient identification	Identification record Disk file
Phase III	Calibration	Computer memory Disk file
Phase IV	Digitizing and contour definition	Computer memory Disk file
Phase V	Data processing and calculation of derived parameters	Computer memory Disk file
Phase VI	Report output	Display screen Printer output Disk file
Phase VII	Data transfer to host	Diskfile on host computer (Main database system)

Figure 2. Data flow diagram.

Table 2. Derived parameter for aortic and pulmonic valve.

Physical quantity		Units	Derived from
Early diastolic velocity	EADV	$m \cdot s^{-1}$	Manual ref. point
Early diastolic gradient	EADG	mmHg	EADV
Mean diastolic velocity	MDV	$m \cdot s^{-1}$	Velocity-time integral
Mean diastolic gradient	MDG	mmHg	Pressure-time integral
End diastolic velocity	EDV	$m \cdot s^{-1}$	Manual ref. point
End diastolic gradient	EDG	mmHg	EDV
Peak systolic velocity	PSV	$m \cdot s^{-1}$	Manual ref. point
Peak systolic gradient	PSG	mmHg	PSV
Mean systolic velocity	MSV	$m \cdot s^{-1}$	Velocity-time integral
Mean systolic gradient	MSG	mmHg	Pressure-time integral
Systolic ejection period	SEP	s^{-3}	Manual ref. point
Diastolic filling period	DFP	s^{-3}	Manual ref. point

because this requires specialized hardware and modification of the Doppler instrument. A semi-automatic system requires less sophisticated and less expensive hardware. The following section describes the different phases of the analysis procedure which starts at the examination of the patient and ends with a clinical record in the main database system of our department (Figs. 2 and 3).

Phase II. Patient identification

The computer-aided analysis starts with the patient identification request. Patient identification data are introduced together with information about the Doppler technique. This part of patient identification, has been expanded with the possibility to minimize part of the input of general patient data such as name, age, etc. by using patient identification number used throughout the hospital. With this number patients general data can be retrieved from the main database which reduces the amount of input at the personal computer for patient identification and at the same time this reference ensures consistency of this data.

Phase III. Calibration

After introduction of patient identification data the user can start the digitizing proces by selecting the part of the trace to be analysed. The first step is the calibration of both the time and velocity scales. The velocity recording can be calibrated in kHz or $m \cdot s^{-1}$. When calibration is done in frequency shift (kHz), it is translated into blood flow velocity, by using the standard Doppler equation:

$$v = \frac{c \cdot f_{max}}{2 \cdot f \cdot \cos \varphi}$$

where c is the velocity of ultrasound in blood $(1560 \, m \cdot s^{-1})$. f_{max} is the maximum frequency shift, f is the transmitted frequency (2.5 MHz) and φ is the angle between the interrogating sound beam and the direction of blood flow.

Table 3. Derived time related parameters.

Physical quantity		Units	Derived from
Pre-ejection period	PEP	s^{-3}	Manual ref. point
RR interval	RR	s^{-3}	Manual ref. point
Heartrate	HR	$bts \cdot min^{-1}$	RR

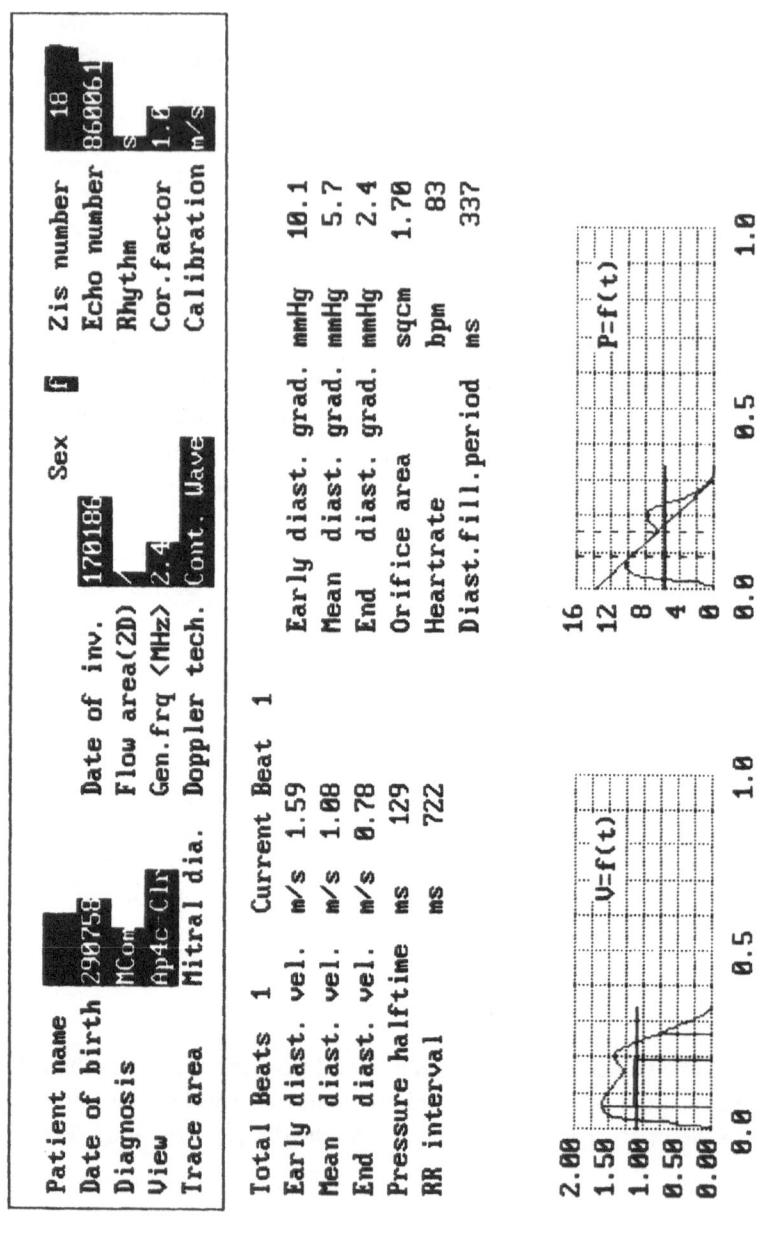

Figure 3.

Phase IV. The digitizing proces and contour definition

The frequency shift of velocity contour is digitized by moving the cursor of the digitizing tablet along the velocity recording. By pressing the cursor button the contour is digitized and simultaneously displayed on the the viewing screen. The system stores the point on the contour where the cursor is at the time of pressing the cursor button as contour point. All points on the contour are subsequently stored until the end of the baseline is entered together with reference points, such as early diastolic velocity, the Q waves of the corresponding and previous QRS complexes of the electrocardiogram. At this moment the system returns to the menu the user has now several options: saving the contour, retracing when not satisfactory or to calculate the specific parameters which are used for clinical decision making.

Phase V. Data processing and calculation of derived parameters

The digitized contours of individual cardiac cycles are stored on a floppy disk which enables us to reconstruct earlier stored contours, and use them for sub-sequent re-analysis. Thus whenever the algorithm of the computer program is optimized or expanded with newly derived parameters, there is no need for retracing the time velocity recording which is time-consuming (and tedious).

Once the contour of a Doppler velocity curve has been stored into the memory of the computer, the program performs an analysis procedure depending upon the valve of which the Doppler trace was recorded (Tables 1, 2 and 3).

Parameter definitions

Early diastolic maximal velocity (EDMV) is defined as the early diastolic peak of the Doppler velocity curve. This velocity over an atrioventricular valve is entered as a reference point on the original tracing.

Early diastolic maximal pressure difference (EDMG) is defined as the early diastolic pressure drop across the atrio-ventricular valve (mitral or tricuspid) area, calculated from early diastolic maximal velocity (EDMV) using the sim-plified Bernoulli equation as proposed by Hatle et al. [1]:

$$(P_1 - P_2) = 4 \times v_2^2 \text{ (mmHg)}$$

where v_2 is Early diastolic maximal velocity (EDMV) in units of $m \cdot s^{-1}$, while the pressure drop is calculated in units of mmHg. P_1 is the atrial pressure, and P_2 is the pressure in the jet where v_2 is measured.

Mean diastolic velocity (MDV) is defined as the mean of maximal instan-taneous velocities throughout diastole.

```
Date 10-08-1985  time 13:26:40
```

```
        - - - DOPPLER REPORT - - -

                    THORAX  CENTER
            ACADEMIC HOSPITAL  DIJKZIGT ROTTERDAM
```

Patientname ▮▮
Date of Birth 22-01-47   Diagnosis   /   Zis number   ▮20524
                            Rhythm   SR   Echo Number 850537
Trace Area   Mitral Dia. Doppler Tech. Cont. Wave   Calibration KHz
View   /   Gen.Frq (MHz) 2.4   Cor.Factor   1.0

BNM	EDV m/s	EDG mmHg	MDV m/s	MDG mmHg	VED m/s	GED mmHg	PHT ms	OA sqcm	RR ms	HR bpm	PEP ms	DFP ms
1	2.41	23.1	1.51	9.8	1.36	7.4	261	0.84	1230	49	60	856
2	2.15	18.6	1.56	10.6	1.67	11.2	274	0.80	1013	39	90	634
3	2.27	20.6	1.46	9.2	1.60	10.2	221	0.99	1163	52	78	815
4	2.36	22.3	1.77	13.2	1.87	14.0	238	0.93	927	65	87	556
5	2.19	19.2	1.67	11.6	1.73	12.0	251	0.88	974	62	68	576
6	2.24	20.1	1.71	13.0	2.08	17.2	308	0.71	781	77	108	415
7	2.16	18.7	1.40	8.5	1.52	9.3	213	1.03	1152	52	76	781
8	2.24	20.0	1.74	12.9	1.88	14.2	240	0.92	900	67	79	506
9	2.41	23.3	1.45	9.6	1.36	7.4	234	0.94	1209	50	62	839
mean	2.27	20.7	1.59	10.9	1.68	11.4	249	0.89	1039	59	79	664
SD	0.10	1.8	0.14	1.8	0.24	3.3	29	0.10	157	9	15	163

Figure 4.

Mean diastolic pressure difference (MDG) is defined as the mean of pressure drops calculated for digitized points during diastole.

End diastolic pressure difference (EDV) is defined as the maximal instantaneous velocity at the onset (Q) of the QRS complex. This point in the cardiac cycle is entered as a reference point by the user [2].

End diastolic pressure difference (EDG) is defined as the pressure drop calculated from the end diastolic velocity (EDV) using the simplified Bernoulli equation.

Pressure halftime $(t_{1/2})$ defined as the time required during diastole for the pressure difference (P_1-P_2) across the (mitral) valve to reduce to onehalf of its maximum value during diastole (EDMG) [3].

Orifice Area (OA) calculated from the pressure halftime using the following equation: $OA = 220/t_{1/2}$ in cm^2 [4, 5].

Data display

Results are displayed on the display screen and their order is dependent upon the valve analyzed. The top of the display screen shows patient identification data together with the examination information. This information can be entered from the keyboard or from a patient identification file which may already be available from previous studies or from the hospitals main database system. The lower part of the screen shows the different parameters derived from one digitized heart beat. Up to 30 beats can be measured in one analysis procedure. At the end of such procedure all individual results as well, the average values of total number of

```
Date 08-10-85 time 13:28:16
---------------------------------------------------------------------------
                         D O P P L E R   R E P O R T
                              Thorax  Center
                    Academic Hospital Rotterdam Dijkzigt
---------------------------------------------------------------------------
Patientname   ■■                              Zis number  ■■20524
Date of Birth 22-01-47    Diagnosis    /      Echo Number 850537
                          Rhythm       SR
Trace Area    Mitral Dia. Doppler Tech. Cont. Wave    Calibration KHz
View          /           Gen.Frq <MHz> 2.4           Cor.Factor  1.0
---------------------------------------------------------------------------
Early diast. Vel.   m/s  2.27  [0.10]  Early diast. Grad.  mmHg   20.7  [ 1.8]
Mean  diast. Vel.   m/s  1.59  [0.14]  Mean  diast. Grad.  mmHg   10.9  [ 1.8]
End   diast. Vel.   m/s  1.68  [0.24]  End   diast. Grad.  mmHg   11.4  [ 3.3]
Pressure Halftime   ms    249  [  29]  Orifice Area        sqcm   0.89  [0.10]
RR interval         ms   1039  [ 157]  Heartrate           bpm      59  [  9]
Pre-Ejec.Period     ms     79  [  15]  Diast.Fill.Period   ms      664  [ 163]
---------------------------------------------------------------------------
All values are mean + SD with n=10
---------------------------------------------------------------------------
Remarks :




---------------------------------------------------------------------------
```

Figure 5.

beats, can be transferred to a disk and a summary report can be printed at any desired moment.

Phase VI. Data reporting

Two different reports are available. The first (Fig. 4) consists of a list of parameters in tabular form containing all individual contour data together with the mean and standard deviation for the total number of contours analyzed. This report is mainly used when information about each individual cardiac cycle is needed. The second report (Fig. 5) consists of a summary of different parameters from the selected analysis procedure, together with the mean and standard deviation. This report can be used for the patient file and can be transferred to the hospitals main data base system. Both reports also have information on patient identification and examination procedure.

Phase VII. Data transfer

A special communication protocol has been developed to transfer the data from the personal computer to the hospitals main database and vice versa. The advantages of this concept are that patient data storage is standardized and centralized. The retrieval of results from the database can be performed by using the main database management system which is already in use for storage and retrieval of data from other investigations. Another feature is that with this protocol the patient identification procedure can be reduced to a minimum because most of this information is already present in the main database. Only a special reference number together with the patients birthdate is used to identify a particular patient.

4. Discussion

Digitization of Doppler echocardiograms is based on both practical considerations and the necessity to reduce random errors due to physiological and methodological factors. These are the inherent large beat-to-beat variability, respiration, cardiac motion during the cardiac cycle and examination technique. It is important for the clinician to have information on the variability when several consecutive beats are analyzed. This is provided by calculating the mean and standard deviation of the beats analyzed. The report contains together with all the information on identification, used Doppler technique, and the results, the information about the variability. This information is helpful for the clinician as it gives an indication on the reliability of the results, for clinical decision making.

Due to the combination of manual input and automated data acquisition, the user has full control over the analysis procedure. At any time during the analysis the user can verify the retrieved or calculated results and decide whether or not he accepts the results or discard them. Only when the data are accepted one can proceed to the next analysis.

Limitations

Inadequate Doppler tracings lead to an underestimation of the maximal velocity and consequently of the pressure drop. Due to manual tracing of the Doppler velocity curve, a scattered digital copy of the original velocity curve will result. For some derived parameters, such as mean diastolic velocity and mean diastolic pressure difference, this will not affect the result, because this error component is averaged. However, for pressure halftime the result depends on the accuracy of the best fitted line, of the downslope of the pressure drop curve, starting with the early diastolic maximal pressure difference: To overcome the previous mentioned problem in this situation an approximating curve is constructed using a least square method, producing a regression line.

Conclusion

This interactive computer program offers both the advantages of manual and automated analysis is a very effective analysis system for Doppler echocardiograms.

References

1. Hatle L, Brubakk A, Tromsdal A, Angelsen B: Noninvasive assessment of pressure drop in mitral stenosis by Doppler ultrasound. Br Heart J 40: 131–140, 1978.
2. Robson DJ, Flaxman JC: Measurement of the end diastolic pressure gradient and mitral valve area in mitral stenosis by Doppler ultrasound. Eur Heart J 5: 660–667, 1984.
3. Hatle L, Angelsen B, Tromsdal A: Noninvasive assessment of atrioventricular pressure halftime by Doppler ultrasound. Circulation 60: 1096–1104, 1979.
4. Dennig K, Rudolph W: Dopplerechokardiographische Bestimmung des Schweregrades der Mitralstenose. Herz 9 (4): 222–230, 1984.
5. Hatle L: Noninvasive assessment of valve lesions with Doppler ultrasound. Herz 9 (4): 213–221, 1984.

II. Color-coded Doppler flow imaging

Two years clinical experience with color-coded real-time two-dimensional Doppler cardiography

Ryozo Omoto, Shunei Kyo, Shinichi Takamoto, Makoto Matsumura,
Yuji Yokote, Koroku Namekawa, Chihiro Kasai, Yoshihiro Yoshikawa
and Akira Koyano

1. Introduction

A noninvasive method for real-time blood-flow Doppler imaging has long been needed in the fields of cardiology and cardiovascular surgery. In 1982, two research groups, Namekawa et al. [1] in Japan and Bommer et al. [2] in the United States, independently described the new technologies of real-time two-dimensional Doppler echocardiography. Namekawa et al., the co-authors of this paper, developed two-dimensional Doppler echocardiography [1, 3] (hereafter abbreviated as 2-D Doppler or color flow mapping) for clinical use, which allows us to obtain intracardiac blood-flow images in real time noninvasively. In April of 1983, the authors first reported [4] on the wide range of clinical applications of real-time two-dimensional Doppler echocardiography using the new device. The authors' group has confirmed the diagnostic effectiveness in acquired valvular disease [5, 6, 7], congenital heart disease [8, 9, 10], and aortic aneurysm [11]. Furthermore, an intraoperative use for various cardiovascular lesions has been found effective [12, 13].

Since the introduction of commercially available 2-D Doppler systems in December of 1983, a number of vigorous studies on color flow mapping have been rapidly carried out in many cardiac centers [14–19]. Regarding the usefulness of a new modality '2-D Doppler', it may be now safely concluded that it provides a dynamic method for studying the spatial distribution of blood flow velocities in the beating heart, unlike any noninvasive or invasive technique previously available [20].

The main purpose of this communication is to describe briefly two years clinical experience with 2-D Doppler in the examinations of acquired valvular diseases, congenital heart diseases and aortic aneurysms at Saitama Medical School.

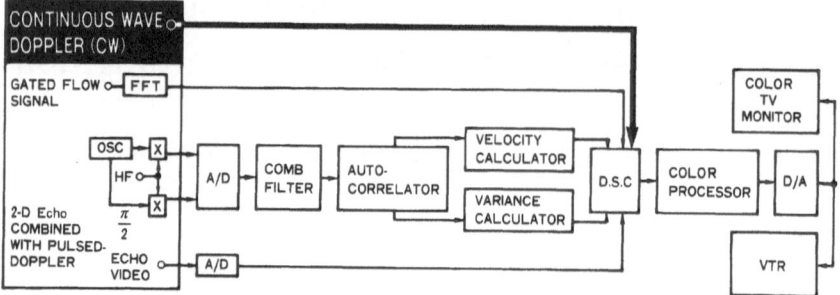

Figure 1. The block diagram of the most recent system (Aloka 880CW); continuous wave Doppler technology is available in this device.

2. 2-D Doppler system

Various types of 2-D Doppler systems were used in two years at Saitama Medical School (Table 1). The block diagram of the most recent system (Aloka-880CW) is shown in Fig. 1. The device combines in principle a conventional pulsed-Doppler system and a newly developed autocorrelator [1, 3], in which blood-flow images within a given cross-section of a beating heart are displayed in real time. The details of the principle and instrumentation are described in a previous paper [3]. Comb filter functions to cancel the effects of wall motions. Only the Doppler signals with low intensity and high velocity can pass throuh the filter as the signals from blood flow. With regard to the direction of blood flow, a red color is given to the blood flowing toward the transducer, while a blue color is given to the blood flowing away from it. The velocity of blood flow is represented by the brightness of each color which is displayed in seven gradations. With regard to the degree of turbulence of blood flow, a green color is added in proportion to the extent of turbulence in sixteen gradations. Therefore, three kinds of information concerning blood flow, the direction, velocity and degree of turbulence are indicated by differences in color. The conventional B-mode echocardiograms are usually superimposed in black and white simultaneously with color-coded blood flow images. M-mode, spectral analysis (fast Fourier transformation, FFT) and continuous wave Doppler (CW) displays are also available with this system. The comparison of sensitivity between FFT filter and color flow filter is shown in Fig.

Table 1. Various systems of 2-D Doppler used clinically in Saitama Group.

Aloka – Initial prototype	from Sept., 1982
– XA 54 (Final prototype)	from Dec., 1982
– 880 (Commercial)	from Dec., 1983
– 880 CW	from Sept., 1984
– XA 340 (Prototype for surface organ)	from Feb., 1985

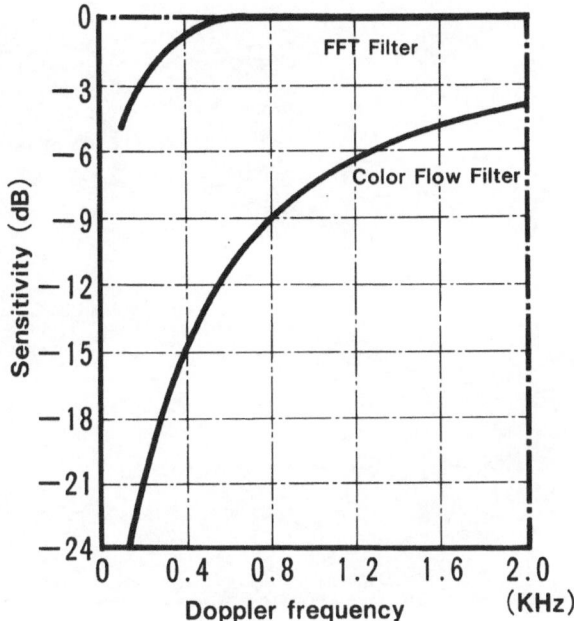

Figure 2. Characteristics of filter sensitivity is compared between FFT filter and color filter.

Table 2. Characteristics of system (Aloka 880 · CW).

Ultrasound frequency	2.5, 3.5 MHz
Pulsed repetion rate	4, 6, 8 MHz
Scanning angle for 2-D Doppler	27.5, 50, 90 degrees
for 2-D echo	90 degrees
Diagnostic range	6, 12, 15, 18, 21 cm
Frame rate	10–30 frames/sec
Display	B-mode, M-mode, FFT, (* * * CW)
Transducer	phased array (13 × 10 mm, 48 elements)
* Maximum detectable flow velocity	* * 120 cm/sec
* Minimum detectable flow velocity	23 cm/sec (B-mode)
	6 cm/sec (M-mode)
Recording	VTR, 35 mm film, instant photo.

* Assuming that beam angle to blood flow is 60 degrees.
* * Images of blood flows with high velocities exceeding this range result in a wrap around of the top portion of Doppler frequencies (aliasing).
* * * Option.

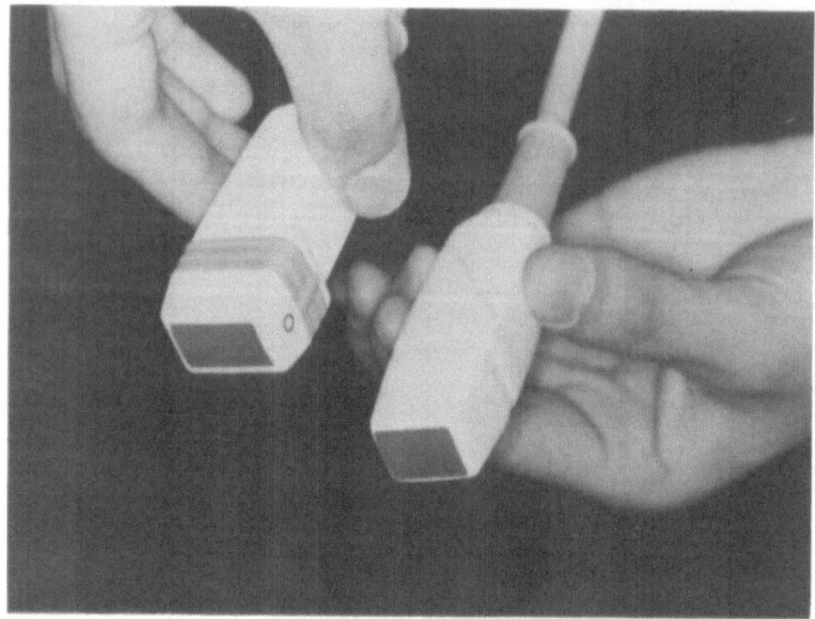

Figure 3. Transducers for a regular color flow mapping (right) and a combined use with CW (left).

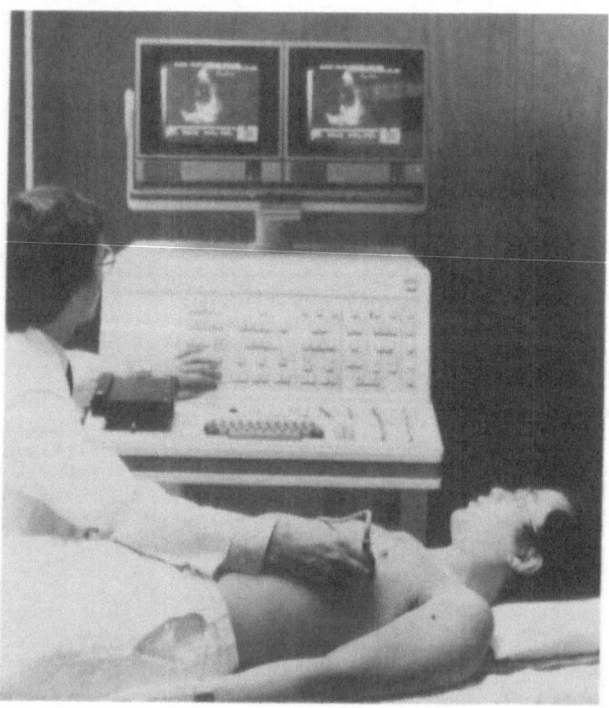

Figure 4. Clinical examination by 2-D Doppler.

2. The sensitivity of color flow filter is slightly (-4 dB at 2 KHz of Doppler frequency) inferior to that of FFT filter. The characteristics of the system are briefly summarized in Table 2. The probe with dual frequency transducer for the combined use of color flow mapping and CW is composed of phased array 48 elements for 2-D imaging (3.5 MHz) and two elements for CW transmitting/receiving (2 MHz). The distance between the center of phased array scanning and the CW elements is 10 mm (Fig. 3). The clinical use of 2-D Doppler system does not require special handling; rather it is used in the same manner as is conventional echocardiography (Fig. 4).

3. Population of the 2-D Doppler examinations

Between September of 1982 and April of 1985, the 2-D Doppler examinations were performed on 2100 patients (pts) with cardiovascular diseases at the department. Among them, the diagnoses of 1035 pts were confirmed by angiography and/or surgery (acquired valvular disease; 432 pts, congenital heart disease; 278 pts, ischemic heart disease; 126 pts, vascular disease; 84, others; 81 pts) (Table 3).

4. Clinical results

4.1 Acquired valvular disease

Evaluation of valvular regurgitation has become the first clinical application using the 2-D Doppler modality. Clinical investigations using 2-D Doppler have shown that it is very useful in the detection of aortic, mitral and tricuspid regurgitations, and that it offers a favorable correlation with angiography or surgical findings in the quantitative evaluation of the severity of the valvular regurgitation [4, 5, 14]. The 2-D Doppler findings in valvular regurgitation show the following distinct

Table 3. Population of 2-D Doppler examination (from September of 1982 to March of 1985).

Disease	No of pts
Valvular HD	423
Ischemic HD	126
Cardiomyopathy	27
Congenital HD	278
Vascular disease	84
Pericardial disease	16
Others	81
Total	1035

characteristics of the Doppler signals: most regurgitant blood flows are characterized as (a) wide-banded and (b) bi-directional flow patterns in spectral analysis. In 2-D Doppler, the regurgitant flow is inlaid with red-and-blue mosaic patterns. We compared the 2-D Doppler findings with the angiography or surgical findings, and set a criteria for the quantitative evaluation of valvular regurgitation. Sellers' classification [4] is used as the criteria for evaluating aortic and mitral regurgitation by angiography. As for the evaluation of tricuspid regurgitation, established diagnosis is made using surgical findings [5], since right ventriculography is not routinely performed in the authors' institute. Prior to the cannulation for cardiopulmonary bypass, the regurgitant jet is examined by a surgeon's forefinger inserted into the right atrium and placed 1 cm above the center of tricuspid valve. The size of the regurgitant jet is compared with the forefinger size and is graded as I (grade 1: smaller than forefinger size in width), II (grade 2: almost same) or III (grade 3: larger). The criteria used for the quantitative evaluation of valvular regurgitation with 2-D Doppler are described in Table 4 (for aortic), Table 5 (for mitral) and Table 6 (for tricuspid). As shown in the tables 2-D Doppler has revealed its sensitive diagnostic capacity in valvular regurgitation and correlated well with cardiac catheterization data. In tricuspid regurgitation, we tend to over-assess by almost one grade compared with the operative evaluation. However, one must take into consideration the time lag

Table 4. Comparison of the grade of aortic regurtitation (AR) assessed by angiography (Angio) and 2-D Doppler (105 ARs). A significant correlation is noted (105 ARs).

Angio \ 2-D Doppler	0°	I°	II°	III°	IV°
0°					
I°	3	18	6		
II°		2	34	8	
III°				21	4
IV°				1	8

The criteria for assessing the severity of AR by 2-D Doppler are based mainly on the maximal distance reached by regurgitant blood-flow images (RFIs) in the left ventricular outflow tract (in long-axis view). I°: RFIs are localized between the region just inferior to the aortic valve and the middle of the level of the anterior mitral leaflet (AML). II°: RFIs reach the level of the tip of AML. III°: RFIs extend to the level of the papillary muscles. IV°: RFIs are visualized deeper and wider beyond the papillary muscles toward the apex.

Table 5. Comparison of the Grade of Mitral Regurgitation (MR) Assessed by Angiocardiography (Angio) and 2-D Doppler (76 MRs). A significant correlation is noted (76 MRs).

Angio \ 2-D Doppler	0°	I°	II°	III°	IV°
0°	////				
I°	1	//9//	2		
II°		1	//28//	4	
III°			2	//21//	2
IV°					//6//

The criteria for assessing the severity of MR by 2-D Doppler are based mainly on the maximal distance reached by regurgitant blood-flow images (RFIs) from the mitral orifice into the left atrium. I°: RFIs are localized immediately posterior to the mitral valve in the left atrium, not extending beyond the middle of the level between the mitral orifice and the ring. II°: RFIs reach almost to the level of the mitral ring. III°: RFIs are present deep, within 2 cm of the level of the mitral ring. IV°: RFIs are present deeper, beyond 2 cm of the level of the mitral ring, and are often visualized diffusely over the entire left attium.

between the 2-D Doppler examination and the operation. Typical 2-D Doppler findings in aortic, mitral and tricuspid regurgitation are shown in Figs. 5, 6 and 7.

Valvular stenosis can be adequately diagnosed with conventional echocardiography by the demonstration of the organic changes causing hemodynamic stenosis. In addition, quantification of pressure gradients across stenotic valves has become available by continuous-wave Doppler ultrasound (CW) [21, 22]. As described above, valvular regurgitation has been demonstrated accurately with 2-D Doppler and found to be highly correlated with the findings of angiography and/or surgery. Hence, it has been suggested that combined use of 2-D Doppler and CW can replace routine cardiac catheterization in some situations, such as where coronary artery lesions are not suspected, or risks of cardiac catheterization are extremely high [23] (Fig. 8).

4.2 Congenital heart disease

The clinical significance of 2-D Doppler in congenital heart disease is that 2-D Doppler can visualize the intracardiac abnormal blood flow in real time. In 278 patients with congenital heart diseases, 2-D Doppler examination was performed (Table 7). Abnormal blood flow with mosaic patterns (shunt flow, regurgitant

Table 6. Comparison of the Grade of Tricuspid Regurgitation (TR) Assessed by Operative Findings (Ope) and 2-D Doppler (50 TRs).

Ope \ 2-D Doppler	0°	I°	II°	III°
0°	░	8	2	
I°		6	8	
II°			11	6
III°				9

Although a significant correlation is noted 2-D Doppler tends to overestimate by almost one grade compared with the operative evaluation. The criteria for assessing the severity of TR by 2-D Doppler are based mainly on the maximal distance reached by regurgitant blood-flow images (RFIs) from the tricuspid valve in the right atrium (in apical four-chamber view) and the presence of significant regurgitant blood flow in the hepatic vein (in subcostal view). I°: RFIs extend half way into the right atrium from the tricuspid valve during systole. II°: RFIs are present diffusely within the entire right atrium. III°: RFIs are present in the entire right atrium. At the same time, significant regurgitant blood flows are demonstrated in the hepatic vein during systole.

flow and/or stenotic flow) was clearly visualized by 2-D Doppler. The diagnoses of these 278 cases were established by cardiac catheterization and/or by surgery. 76 cases of corrective surgery and 12 cases of palliative procedure were performed after full examination with both 2-D Doppler and cardiac catheterization. In 6 cases of these 88 cases (6.8%), we could not obtain diagnostic information by 2-D Doppler. In other 3 cases (3.4%) we could obtain diagnostic information by 2-D Doppler. However, it was not satisfactory to perform a corrective surgery, because we could not detect the azygos connection and the persistent left superior vena cava in one case of cor triatrium with VSD and also we could not detect the associated partial anomalous pulmonary venous connection in two cases of ASD. Therefore, in 79 cases (89.8%) we could obtain satisfactory diagnostic information for surgery by 2-D Doppler diagnosis which was consistent with catheterization diagnosis. 2-D Doppler has been found to be also very useful for determing good timing of palliative shunt surgery and in evaluating the effectiveness of shunt surgery, because 2-D Doppler is absolutely noninvasive and can be performed repeatedly. It is suggested that surgery can be carried out without cardiac catheterization in significant number of congenital heart diseases.

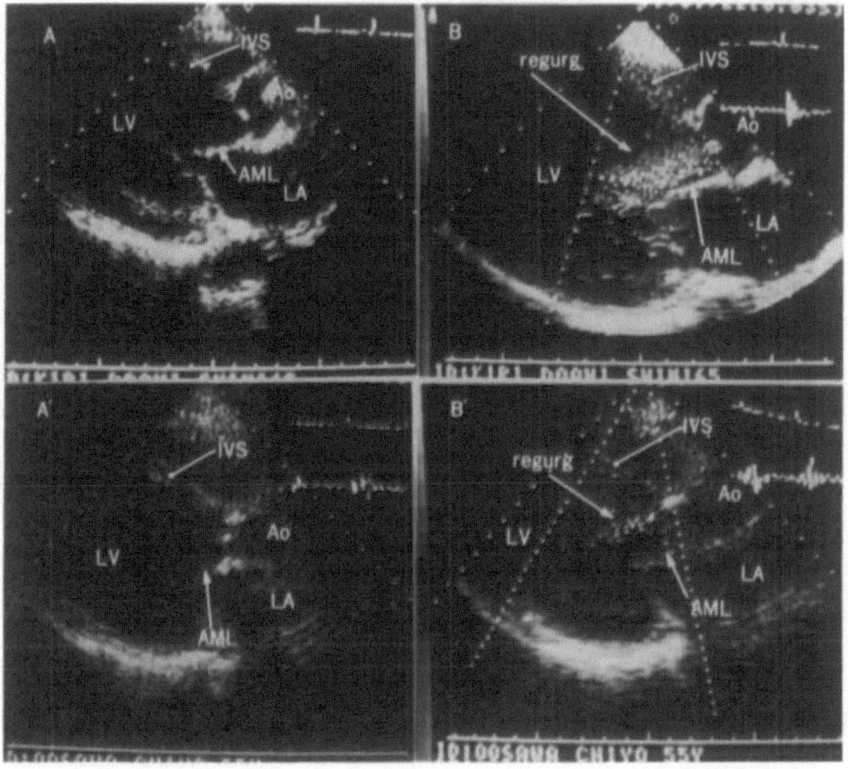

Figure 5. 2-D Doppler images in two patients with Sellers' grade 3 and grade 2 aortic regurgitations. A: B-mode (grade 3). B: 2-D Doppler (ditto). A': B-mode (grade 2). B': 2-D Doppler (ditto). AML: anterior mitral leaflet, regurg: regurgitation.

4.3 Aortic aneurysm

2-D Doppler examination was performed in 26 abdominal aortic aneurysms and 33 dissecting aortic aneurysms (10 type-A pts and 23 type-B pts). In abdominal aortic aneurysms, 2-D Doppler findings were completely compatible with angiographical findings (Table 8). In dissecting aortic aneurysm, however, diagnostic effectiveness seems to be so far rather poor (Table 9). Dissecting aortic aneurysm frequently involves the thoracic and abdominal aorta widely and it is very difficult to obtain the entire image of the whole diseased aorta by conventional echography due to the narrow beam window as shown in our data of Table 9. Intraoperative scanning of 2-D Doppler gives almost complete three-dimensional information about the structure and the blood flow very easily. The operation for dissecting aortic aneurysm is mainly aimed at closure of the entry and relacement of the dilated aorta and leaves large parts of the dissected aorta in situ. Therefore, it is very important to confirm that blood flow in the remnant aorta to the vital

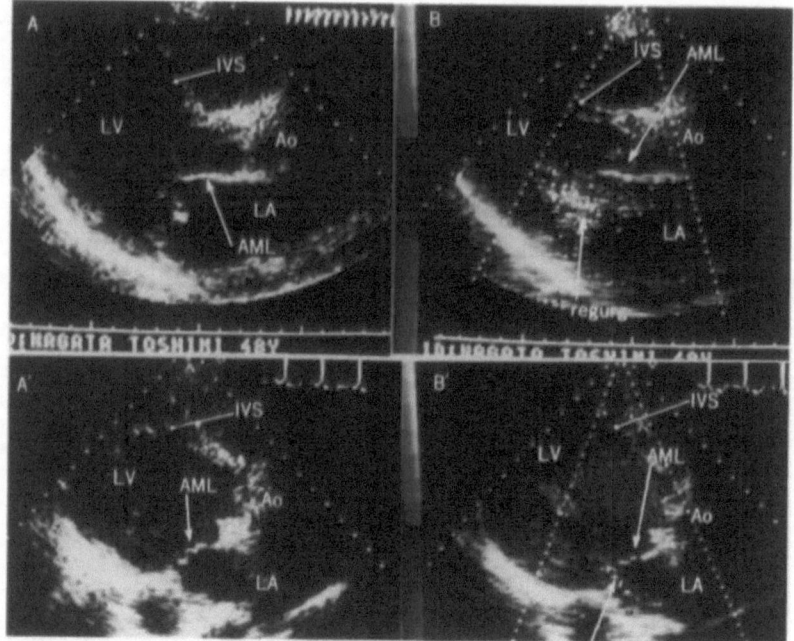

Figure 6. 2-D Doppler images in two patients with Sellers' grade 3 and grade 2 mitral regurgitations.
A: B-mode (grade 3). B: 2-D Doppler (ditto). A': B-mode (grade 2). B': 2-D Doppler (ditto); Lower
arrow shows regurgitant jet in the left atrium in systole.

organs is well reestablished after the operative procedure. Usefulness of intraoperative 2-D Doppler in dissecting aortic aneurysm was demonstrated clinically
[12, 13] (Fig. 9).

4.4 New techniques; 7.5 MHz linear transducer and transesophageal approach

One of limitations of 2-D Doppler technology is its poor ability in visualization of
blood flow with low velocity in a small vessel like a coronary artery. With 7.5 MHz
linear transducer, coronary arteries were often visualized during surgery by 2-D
Doppler (Fig. 10). A saphenous vein graft for aorto-coronary bypass is visualized
much easier than native coronary artery.

An endoscopic probe for color flow mapping by a transesophageal approach
has been recently used clinically to evaluate the clinical effectiveness in cardiac
surgical patients. The transducer of the probe is a phased array type with 5 MHz
ultrasound frequency. It is suggested that the transesophageal approach of 2-D
Doppler is useful for the imediate evaluation of surgical procedure as the intraoperative use of 2-D Doppler with a standard flow mapping probe. Transesophageal approach does not interrupt surgical procedures for color flow map-

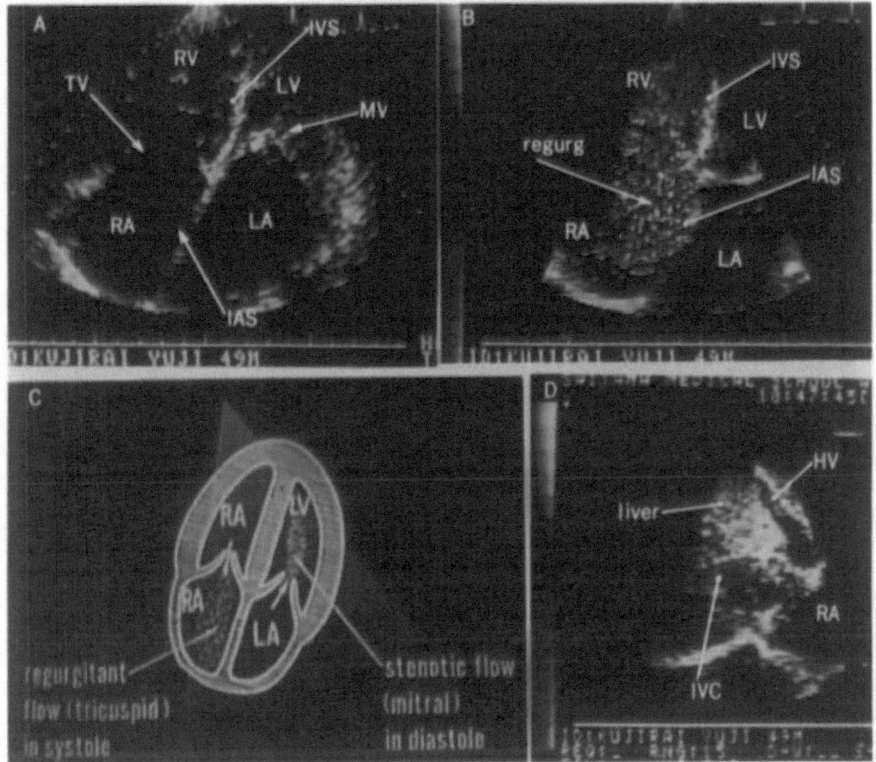

Figure 7. 2-D Doppler images in a patient with grade 3 tricuspid regurgitation. A: B-mode. B: 2-D Doppler; Mosaic patterns are seen in the right atrium in systole. C: Schematic representation. D: 2-D Doppler image of liver; Regurgitant flow into hepatic vein is displayed in red color in systole. HV: hepatic vein.

ping. An improvement in sensitivity of color flow mapping seems to be required for further application of endoscopic-type small transducers.

5. Conclusions

The conclusions in this communication are summarized as follows:
1. 2-D Doppler has been successfully developed for wide clinical application.
2. 2-D Doppler has been found very useful in detecting and estimating quantitatively the degree of valvular regurgitation.
3. Combined use of 2-D Doppler and continuous-wave Doppler (CW) has been effective in evaluating quantitatively stenotic valvular lesions.
4. It has been suggested that combined use of 2-D Doppler and CW may replace routine cardiac catheterization in some situations, such as where coronary

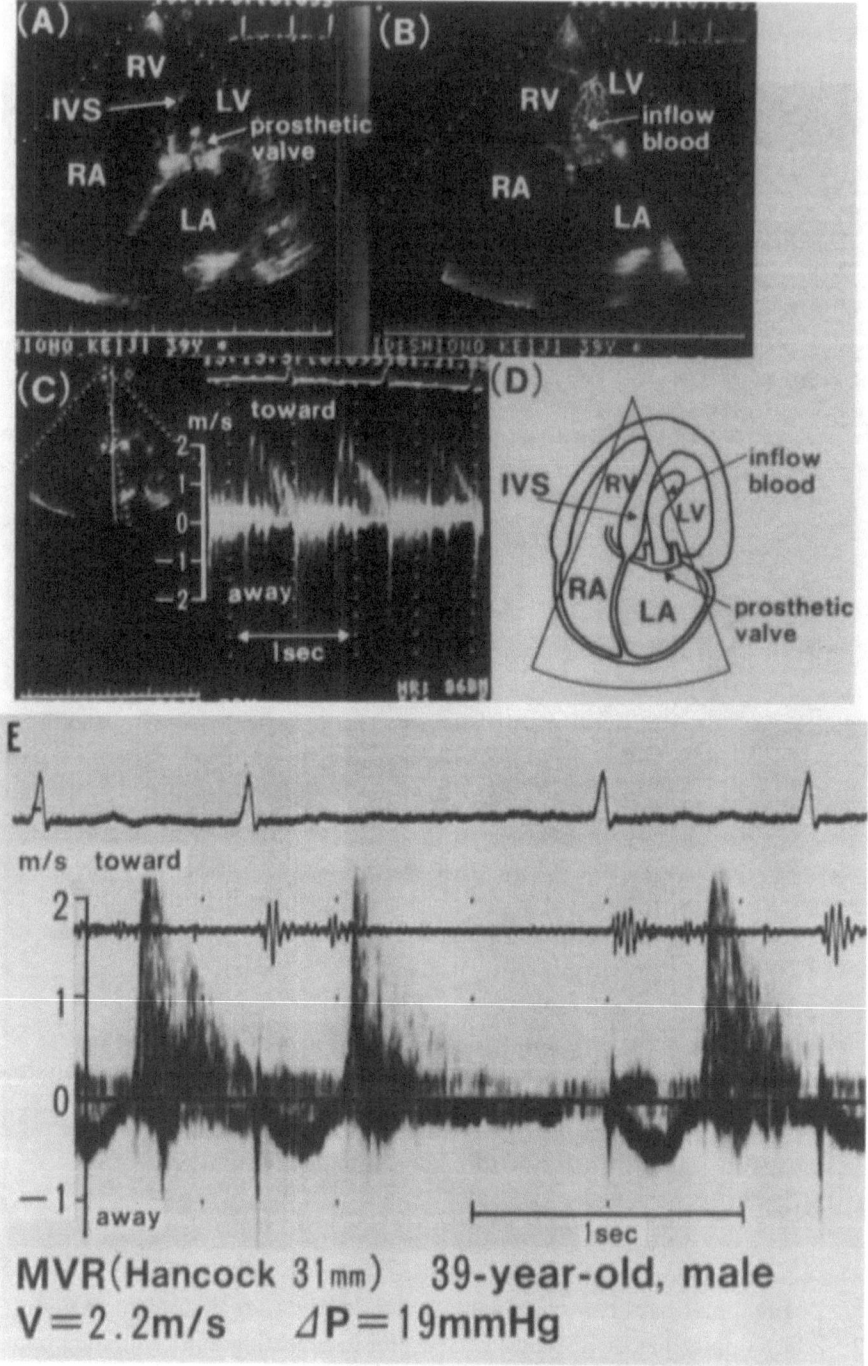

Figure 8. Combined use of 2-D Doppler and CW in a patient with mitral prosthetic valve (Hancock). A: B-mode (Apical four-chamber view). B: 2-D Doppler; Inflow blood is turbulent and directed toward interventricular septum (IVS). C: Display by the combined use. Peak velocity across mitral prosthetic valve in diastole is 2.2 m/sec. Pressure gradient ($\triangle p$) is calculated as below: $\triangle p = 4 \times (2.2)^2 = 19$ (mmHg). Increase in pressure gradient may indicate prosthetic valve failure. D: Schematic representation. E: Strip-chart recording of CW Doppler signals for measurement of maximum velocity.

Table 7. Population of 2-D Doppler examination in congenital heart diseases.

Diseases	Under 15-year-old	Over 15-year-old	Total
ASD	37	38	75
VSD	62	15	76
TOF	18	15	23
TGA	12	0	12
PDA	20	3	23
PS, PA	12	1	13
ECD	9	4	13
Others	33	10	43
Total	202	76	278

Table 8. Result of 2-D Doppler examination in 26 abdominal aortic aneurysms (AAA).

* Blood flow visualization	26/26
* Re-entry of dissection	2/2
* Disruption site of anastomosis aneurysm	1/1

Table 9. Results of 2-D Doppler examination in 33 dissecting aortic aneurysms (DAA).

(1)	Differentiation between true and false lumens	24/33 (73%)
(2)	Visualization of aortic blood flow	
	Thoracic Ao	19/33 (58%)
	Abdominal Ao	28/33 (85%)
(3)	Confirmation of entry site	
	Type A	3/10 (30%)
	Type B	3/23 (13%)

artery lesions are suspected, or risks of cardiac catheterization are extremely high.

5. 2-D Doppler has been found a useful noninvasive diagnostic tool for congenital heart diseases, particularly useful for the evaluation of the severity of the disease. Under special circumstances, when a patient is critically ill, for instance, 2-D Doppler findings alone may decide the indication for cardiac surgery without examination by cardiac catheterization.

6. In dissecting aortic aneurysm diagnostic effectiveness of 2-D Doppler is so far limited. However, intraoperative use of 2-D Doppler in the surgery of dissecting aortic aneurysm seems to be most promising.

7. New techniques with the 7.5 MHz linear transducer and the endoscopic transesophageal approach also seem promising.

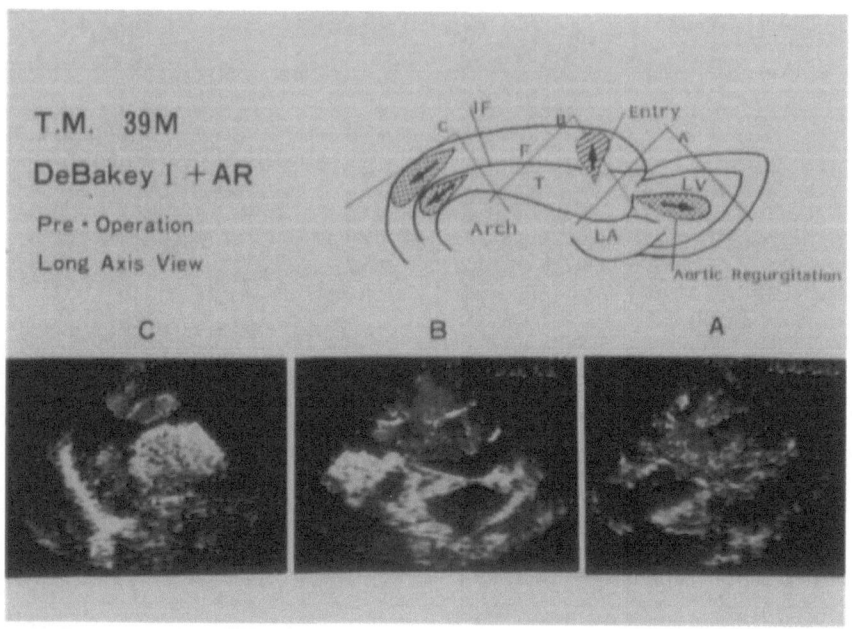

Figure 9. Intraoperative use of 2-D Doppler in DeBakey type-1 dissecting aortic aneurysm.

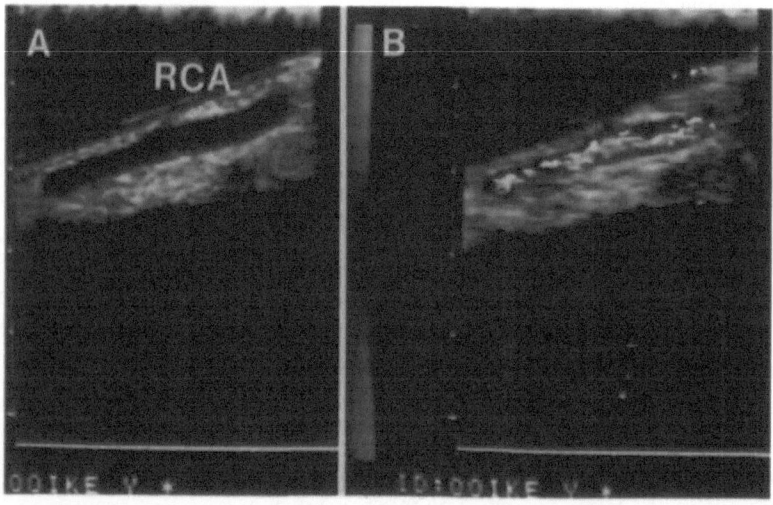

Figure 10. Visualization of a right coronary artery (RCA) during coronary bypass surgery 7.5 MHz linear flow mapping probe is used.

References

1. Namekawa K, Kasai C, Tsukamoto M, Koyano A: Imaging of blood flow using autocorrelation. Ultrasound in Medicine & Biology 8 (Supp.): 138, 1982.
2. Bommer W, Miller L: Real-time two-dimensional color-flow Doppler: Enhanced Doppler flow imaging in the diagnosis of cardiovascular disease (Abstract). Am J Cardiol 49: 944, 1982.
3. Kasai C, Namekawa K, Koyano A, Omoto R: Real-time two-dimensional flow mapping using auto-correlation. In: Kaveh, M et al. (eds) Acoustic Imaging, Vol. 13. Plenum Publishing Corporation, 1984.
4. Omoto R, Yokote Y, Takamoto S, Tamura F, Asano H, Namekawa K, Kasai C, Tsukamoto M, Koyano A: Clinical significance of newly developed real-time intracardiac two-dimensional blood flow imaging system (2-D Doppler). Jpn Circ J 47: 974, 1983.
5. Omoto R (ed.): Color atlas of real-time two-dimensional Doppler echocardiography. Shindan-To-Chiryosha (Tokyo) (delivered by Lea & Febiger, Philadelphia), 1984.
6. Omoto R, Yokote Y, Takamoto S, Kyo S, Ueda K, Asano H, Namekawa K, Kasai C, Kondo Y, Koyano A: The development of real-time two-dimensional Doppler echocardiography and its clinical significance in acquired valvular diseases with special reference to the evaluation of valvular regurgitation. Jpn Heart J 25: 325–340, 1984.
7. Omoto R, Yokote Y, Takamoto S, Ueda K, Emoto H, Hasegawa K, Tamura F, Asano H: Quantitative evaluation of valvular regurgitation in aortic, mitral and tricuspid regurgitation with '2-D Doppler', Jpn Circ J 48: 768–769, 1984.
8. Kyo S, Takamoto S, Ueda K, Emoto H, Tamura F, Asano H, Yokote Y, Omoto R, Takanawa E: Clinical significance of newly developed real-time two-dimensional Doppler echocardiography (2-D Doppler) in congenital heart diseases with special reference to the assessment of the intracardiac shunts. Proceedings of the 43rd Meeting of Japan Society of Ultrasonics in Medicine, pp. 465–466, 1983.
9. Kyo S, Omoto R, Takamoto S, Takanawa E: Clinical significance of color flow mapping real-time two-dimensional Doppler echocardiography (2-D Doppler) in congenital heart disease (Abstract). Circulation 70: II–37, 1984.
10. Kyo S, Omoto R, Takamoto S, Yokote Y: Noninvasive analysis of bi-directional multi-phasic intracardiac shunts by real-time two-dimensional Doppler echocardiography (Abstract). Circulation 70: II–365, 1984.
11. Asano H, Takamoto S, Kyo S, Ueda K, Emoto H, Yamada I, Yokote Y, Omoto R: Clinical assessment of the aortic disease by real-time two-dimensional Doppler Echocardiography. Proceedings of the 43rd Meeting of Japan Society of Ultrasonics in Medicine, pp. 171–172, 1983.
12. Takamoto S, Kondo Y, Yoshikawa Y, Kasai C, Koyano A, Kyo S, Yokote Y, Omoto R: The first clinical experiences of intra-operative real-time two-dimensional Doppler echocardiography in the disserting aneurysm of the aorta, J. Ultrasound in Medicine 3 (Suppl.): 167, 1984.
13. Takamoto S, Adachi H, Matsumura M, Yokote Y, Omoto R: Intraoperative color flow mapping by real-time two-dimensional Doppler echocardiography for evaluation of valvular and congenital heart diseases, and vascular disease. Read at the 65th Annual Meeting of the American Association for Thoracic Surgery, April 29, 1985.
14. Miyatake K, Okimoto M, Kinoshita N, Izumi S, Owa M, Takao S, Sakakibara H, Nimura Y: Clinical applications of a new type of real-time two-dimensional Doppler flow imaging system. Am J Cardiol 54: 857–868, 1984.
15. Sahn DJ, Swensson RE, Valdes-Cruz LM, Scagnelli S, Main J: Two-dimensional color flow mapping for evaluation of ventricular septal defect shunts: A new diagnostic modality (Abstract). Circulation 70: II–364, 1984.
16. Yock PH, Segal J, Teirstein PS, Schnittger I, Popp RL: Doppler color flow mapping: utility in valvular regurgitation (Abstract). Circulation 70: II–38, 1984.
17. Sewart WJ, Levine RA, King ME, Main J: Inital experience with color-coded two-dimensional

Doppler echocardiography (Abstract). Circulation 70: II–405, 1984.

18. Yoshikawa J, Kato H, Yoshida K, Asaka T, Yanagihara K, Okumachi F, Shiratori K, Koizumi K: Real-time two-dimensional Doppler echocardiographic diagnosis of aortic regurgitation in the presence of a mitral prosthesis (Abstract). Circulation 70: II–39, 1984.

19. Sahn DJ, Valdes-Cruz L, Scagnelli S, Tomizuka F, Elias W, Covell J: Two-dimensional Doppler color flow mapping for spatial localization and quantitation of aortic insufficiency: Validation of a new diagnostic modality using an open chest animal model (Abstract). Circulation 70: II–38, 1984.

20. Sahn DJ: Real-time two-dimensional Doppler echocardiographic flow mapping. Circulation 71: 849–853, 1953.

21. Hatle J, Brubakk A, Tromsdol A, Angelsen B: Noninvasive assessment of pressure drop in mitral stenosis by Doppler ultrasound. Br Heart J 40: 131–140, 1978.

22. Hatle L, Angelson B, Tromsdol A: Noninvasive assessment of aortic stenosis by Doppler ultrasound. Br Heart J 43: 284–292, 1980.

23. Omoto R, Yokote Y, Takamoto S, Kyo S, Asano H, Matsumura M, Kasai C, Namekawa K, Miura K, Kondo Y: Clinical significance of combined use of color flow mapping and continuous-wave Doppler in acquired vascular diseases. Proceedings of the 3rd International Cardiac Doppler Symposium (San Diego), 1985.

Two-dimensional Doppler flow mapping in adult cardiology: advantages and limitations

Paul G. Yock, Ingela Schnittger and Richard L. Popp

Introduction

Adult echocardiographers have been slower than their pediatric colleagues to enthusiastically endorse two-dimensional 'color-flow' Doppler echocardiography (2D-Doppler). At least in the United States we are still debating whether 2D-Doppler offers significant practical advantages over the 'conventional' pulsed and continuous wave Doppler techniques (V-mode*) in adult patients. The purpose of this review is to examine the advantages and limitations of 2D-Doppler as applied to some of the diagnostic problems which are common in adult cardiology. The usefulness of 2D-Doppler in congenital disease is extensively reviewed by the pediatric cardiology contributors in this volume; accordingly this section will focus on the assessment of stenotic and regurgitant valvular lesions in native and prosthetic valves, applications to ischemic heart disease and the potential usefulness of 2D-Doppler in noninvasive measurement of cardiac output. Throughout this discussion 2D-Doppler will be compared to current pulsed/continuous wave V-mode techniques; however, it is important to emphasize that 2D- and V-mode Doppler should be regarded as complementary modalities in an integrated cardiac ultrasound examination.

Stenotic valve lesions

Estimation of transvalvular pressure gradients based on Doppler velocity measurements is the most useful overall application of V-mode Doppler echocardiographic methods in an adult population. The quantitative measurement of high velocities is not readily accomplished by 2D-Doppler systems alone. These

---

* In the absence of an accepted convention, 'V-mode' will be used here to refer to conventional pulsed and continuous wave Doppler velocity recordings based on a single ultrasound beam.

systems alias* at relatively low velocities, effectively precluding accurate velocity measurements in stenotic jets. In favorable cases aliasing may produce multiple layers within the flow stream on the 2D images, enabling the operator to estimate the approximate velocity range. The commercially available Aloka system** combines continuous wave V-mode capability with 2D-Doppler imaging using the same transducer, allowing convenient switching between the two modalities, so that high velocities can be easily measured.

Although V-mode velocity determinations are more directly useful than 2D-Doppler in quantitating valvular stenosis, the V-mode method suffers in principle from inability to determine the true axis of jet flow. According to the Doppler equation, if there is an angle deviation theta between the ultrasound beam and the axis of flow, the velocity will be underestimated by an amount proportional to cosine theta. Concern over beam/flow deviation led to initial attempts to 'angle correct' V-mode signals for the presumed direction of jet flow based on the appearance of the valves, chambers or vessels on the 2D echocardiographic study. Unfortunately, predicting the axis of flow from the anatomic image required a high degree of clairvoyance. More recently, investigators have begun to rely on aspects of the Doppler V-mode signal itself to optimize beam/flow orientation. Hatle has suggested that a relatively strong distribution of high-velocity components in a continuous wave signal is a indirect indication of favorable alignment; she points out, however, that this strategy is by no means infallible [1].

The uncertainty concerning beam/flow angle deviation has led in practice to a 'shotgun' strategy of imaging high velocity flows with V-mode instruments: jets are recorded from multiple windows on the chest, and the highest velocity signal is taken as representing the best beam/flow alignment. This strategy is particularly relevant in the case of aortic stenosis, where the jet orientation may be quite variable and any one of several transducer positions – apex, suprasternal or right/left parasternal interspaces – may yield the optimal velocity signal. Given a skilled operator, the 'shotgun' method is actually quite efficient and correlations with data from the catheterization laboratory for pressure gradients across all four valves have been excellent.

The development of 2D-Doppler offers the potential for a still more expeditious and perhaps more reliable approach to the problem of beam/flow deviation. Given an instrument with combined 2D-Doppler and V-mode capabilities, one of two approaches is possible: (a) The transducer is placed in a position in which the optimal jet is imaged by 2D-Doppler. The V-mode signal can then be recorded,

---

* Doppler systems based on pulsed wave transmission can only record velocities up to a certain limit; above this limit velocities appear to abruptly change phase, or direction, by 180° in a phenomenon known as 'aliasing.'

** Aloka system 880, Tokyo, Japan. (Distribution in the U.S. by Johnson & Johnson Ultrasound, Irex Group, Ramsey, N.J.)

the deviation between the V-mode cursor and the apparent axis of flow on 2D-Doppler noted, and the velocity corrected by cosine theta (Plate 1): (b) The appearance of the jet on the 2D-Doppler image can be used as a guide to optimally position the V-mode beam effectively parallel to flow.

Recently Nakagawa *et al.* compared the second 2D-Doppler strategy with the conventional V-mode technique in estimating transmitral gradients in 41 patients with mitral stenosis [2]. In their hands the V-mode method showed a tendency to underestimate valve gradients and correlated less well with catheterization data than the 2D-Doppler guided velocity measurements ($r = 0.96$ versus 0.91). The beam direction in the V-mode method was shown to deviate up to 40 degrees from the angle of flow indicated by 2D-Doppler (cosine $40 = 0.77$, leading to a 23% underestimation of velocity).

Two potential problems with the use of 2D-Doppler for beam/flow alignment must be mentioned. First, the 2D-Doppler image contains information about flow only in the plane of the image; the azimuthal or 'z' axis is not taken into account, so that some underestimation of flow velocity is still expected. A second and more practical limitation is that in some cases stenotic jets are difficult to image, presumably due in part to problems with sensitivity (see below). In our experience this seems to be particularly true in the case of aortic stenosis, where problems of beam/flow deviation might be expected to be the most severe.

Whether or not use of 2D-Doppler for jet orientation proves to be advantageous in a particular laboratory setting will also depend on the relative expertise of the operators with V-mode and 2D-Doppler. At a minimum it seems reasonable that the ability to confirm jet orientation by 2D-Doppler may provide a useful quality control check for laboratories doing quantitative gradient estimation by V-mode Doppler.

Regurgitant valve lesions

While V-mode Doppler has proven extremely sensitive in the detection of regurgitant lesions, efforts to quantitate the severity of regurgitation are still being refined. Two basic strategies are evolving. The first uses Doppler data along with 2D echocardiographic images to estimate total versus effective anterograde stroke volumes across a regurgitant valve. Although this set of techniques is promising, it involves a moderate amount of 'off-line' processing effort and is subject to the same errors which have plagued volume determinations by 2D echocardiography and cardiac output measurements by Doppler.

A second strategy involves 'mapping' the extent of the regurgitant jet using pulsed wave Doppler. In this method the Doppler sample volume is used to explore the limits of the regurgitant jet, mapping the perimeter at which the regurgitant velocity signals are no longer detectable above noise. In general, low volume regurgitant jets tend to dissipate near the valve, while the jets from severe

72

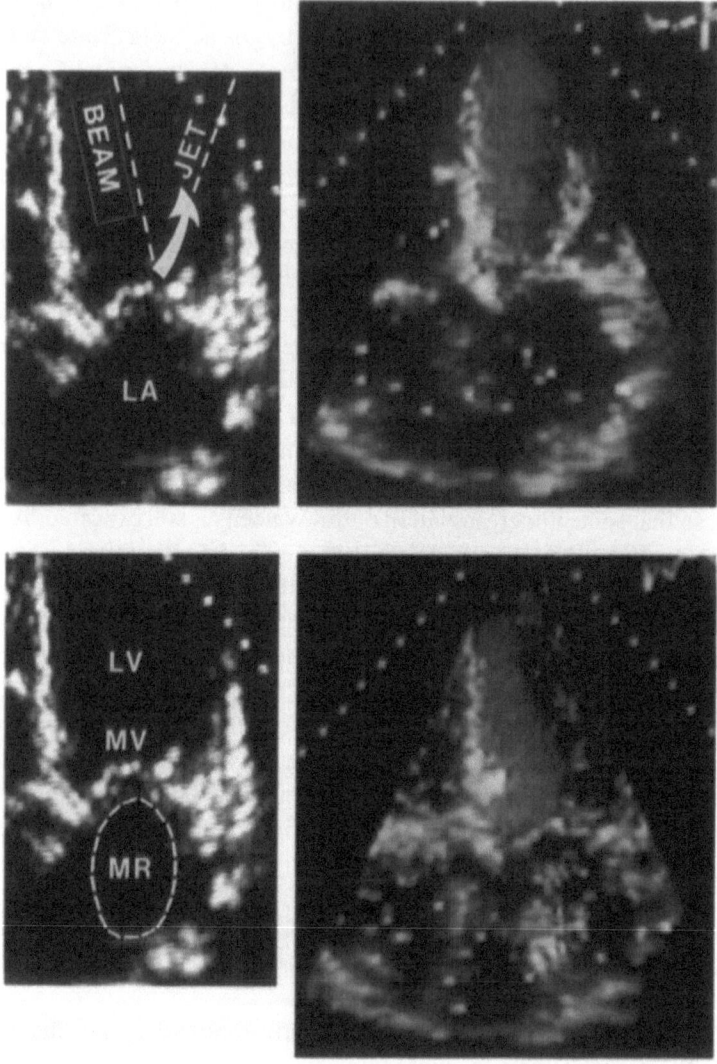

Plate 1. 2D-Doppler images of mitral stenosis and mitral regurgitation in the same patient (Aloka instrument). Corresponding two-dimensional echocardiographs are presented at the left of the color flow images for reference. *Top:* the orange jet of mitral stenosis is directed into the lateral portion of the ventricle in this 2D-Doppler image. If a V-mode recording was made from the same transducer position, the beam axis would deviate from the true axis of flow as indicated by the dashes lines. LA = left atrium. *Bottom:* mitral regurgitation (MR) appears as a 'mosaic' or confetti-like pattern in the left atrium. LV = left ventricle, MV = mitral valve.

lesions extend deeply into the 'upstream' chamber (Fig. 1). The mapping method, originally described by Abbasi *et al.* [3], is conceptually straightforward, requires no 'off-line' operator time and has been shown to correlate fairly well with angiographic estimates of the severity of regurgitation [3–5]. However, the method is relatively time-consuming and no doubt there is wide inter-operator variability depending on the skill and patience of the individual performing the examination.

Two-dimensional Doppler is eminently well suited for mapping analysis and it is this application, above all, which has brought 2D-Doppler to the attention of adult cardiologists. The capacity for real-time 2D display of the regurgitant jet velocity profile has immediate visual appeal due to its resemblance to familiar angiographic images. A well-imaged regurgitant jet (Plates 2, 3) is recognizable to anyone who has experience with angiography or contrast echocardiography. On the other hand, the appearance of regurgitant lesions with 2D-Doppler can be subtle in some cases, with a faint 'sprinkle' of confetti or mosaic-like signals representing the jet (Plate 1). A good deal of operator experience is necessary to maximize the detection of these flows by means of optimal transducer positioning as well as instrument setting (gain, velocity limits, etc). It is not uncommon in laboratories with established expertise in conventional V-mode Doppler that the 2D-Doppler initially misses some regurgitant jets detected by V-mode instruments.

The initial Stanford experience with 2D-Doppler in the assessment of valvular regurgitation is probably representative in this respect. We studied 46 patients with known regurgitation using both V-mode and 2D-Doppler techniques [6]. The 2D-Doppler studies were performed following the V-mode examinations by the same operator in order to bias the study in favor of detecting regurgitant jets by 2D-Doppler. Nevertheless, when compared to angiography, 2D-Doppler was somewhat less sensitive than conventional V-mode Doppler in detecting mitral and aortic regurgitation (Fig. 2). Other investigators have reported higher sen-

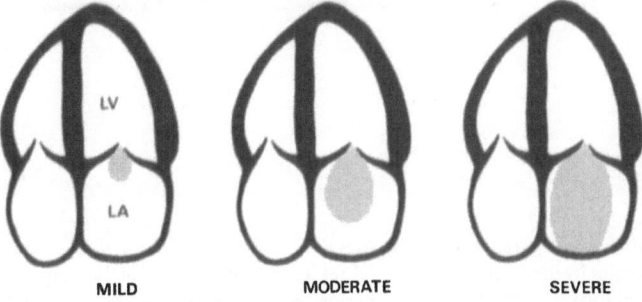

MILD   MODERATE   SEVERE

Figure 1. Schematic depicting mapping analysis for mitral regurgitation. With mild regurgitation, jet velocities are detected near the valve only. When regurgitation is severe, jet velocities can be mapped to the posterior atrial wall. LV = left ventricle, LA = left atrium.

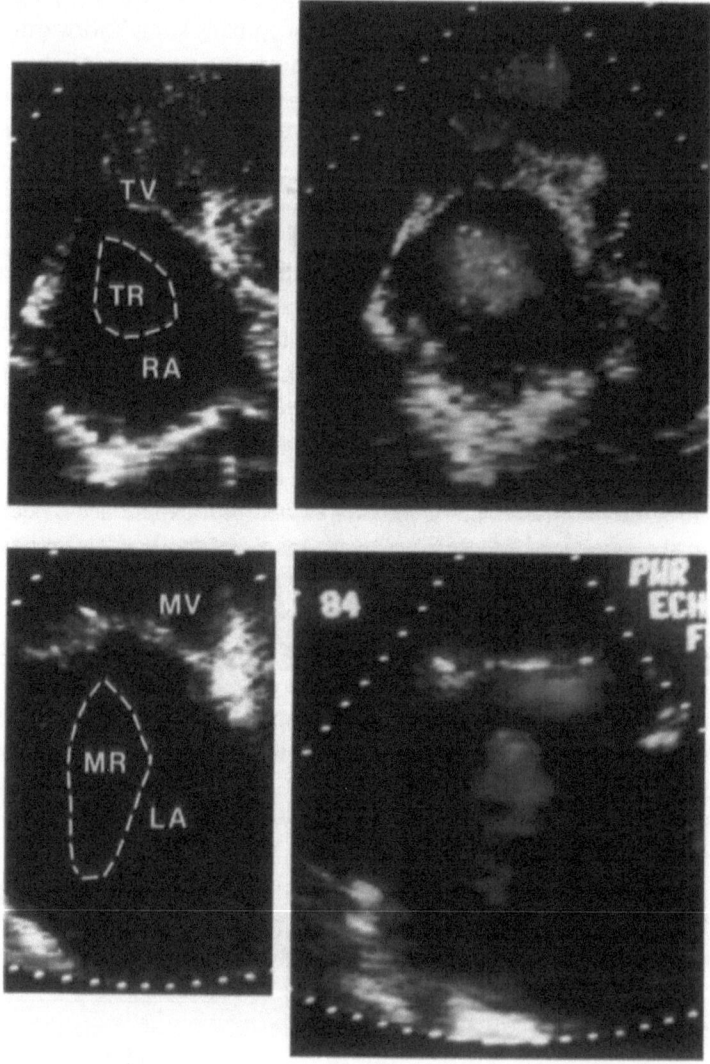

Plate 2. Top: tricuspid regurgitation (TR), Aloka 2D-Doppler. Flow away from the transducer is assigned a blue color by this instrument. The TR jet comes into the plane of the image a short distance from the tricuspid valve (TV). RA = right atrium. *Bottom:* mitral regurgitation (MR), Acoustec 2D-Doppler. The color convention is opposite to Aloka: flow away from the transducer (i.e., the MR jet) is red. The blue patch may represent motion of the valve tissue itself, or aliasing of a portion of the MR signal (see text). LA = left atrium, MV = mitral valve.

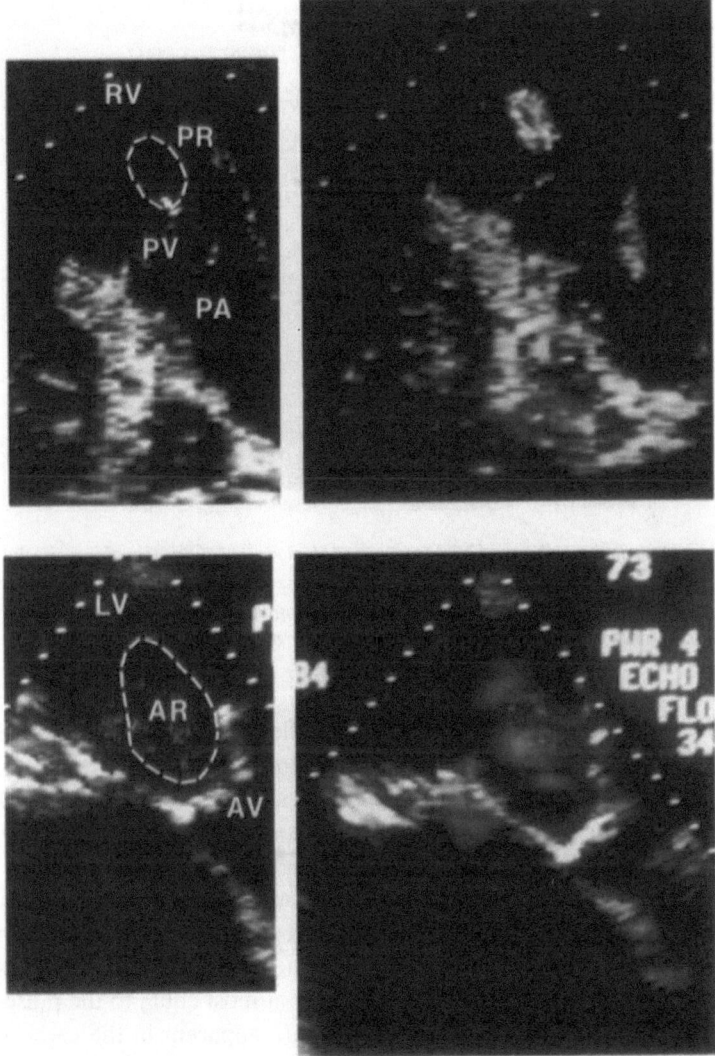

Plate 3. Top: pulmonic regurgitation (PR), Aloka 2D-Doppler. The characteristic 'flame' of pulmonic regurgitation originates at the pulmonic valve leaflets (PV). RV = right ventricle, PA = pulmonary artery. *Bottom:* aortic regurgitation (AR), Acoustec 2D-Doppler. The predominant color is blue, indicating flow toward the transducer. Patches of red within the AR jet are caused by aliasing of the high velocity signals. LV = left ventricle; AV = aortic valve.

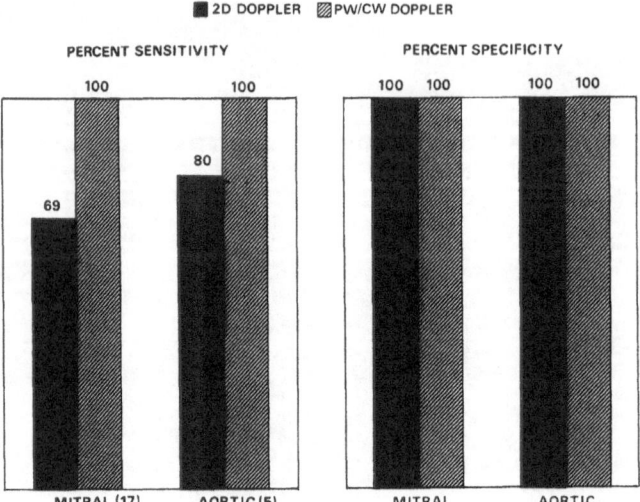

Figure 2. Sensitivity and specificity of 2D-Doppler and V-mode (PW/CW) Doppler in the detection of aortic and mitral regurgitation. Of 46 patients studied with regurgitation of one or more valves, 17 had mitral regurgitation and 5 had aortic regurgitation by angiography. Percent sensitivity and specificity data shown here are relative to angiographic findings. See text for details.

sitivity data [7], and no doubt our findings reflect, in part, the influence of the extended learning curve in the use of this technique. In addition to the experience factor, however, our data clearly indicate that there was a relative lack of sensitivity in the prototype 2D-Doppler instrument we tested compared to the conventional V-mode instrument used.* When the dimensions of the signal perimeter map determined by conventional V-mode pulsed-wave mapping techniques were compared with the dimensions of the 2D-Doppler map generated from the same transducer position, a clear trend emerged: the perimeters of the 2D-Doppler maps were generally less than, or at most equal to the pulsed wave perimeters (Fig. 3). This discrepancy was more apparent in the case of mitral regurgitation than in aortic regurgitation, perhaps because the perimeters of the mitral regurgitant jet are located farther from the transducer in an apical view and thus attenuation may be more significant.

The relative lack of sensitivity with increasing depth of the 2D-Doppler tested in our initial series may help explain the somewhat weaker correlation we found in comparing it with V-mode Doppler against angiographic grading of regurgitation (Fig. 4). Theses findings are useful in highlighting one essential technical feature of imaging with 2D-Doppler: given the limited sensitivity of 2D-Doppler with depth, the adult examination must be modified to place the transducer as close as possible to the flow region of interest. Nonstandard views of the atrio-

---

* Irex Exemplar, Ramsey, N.J.

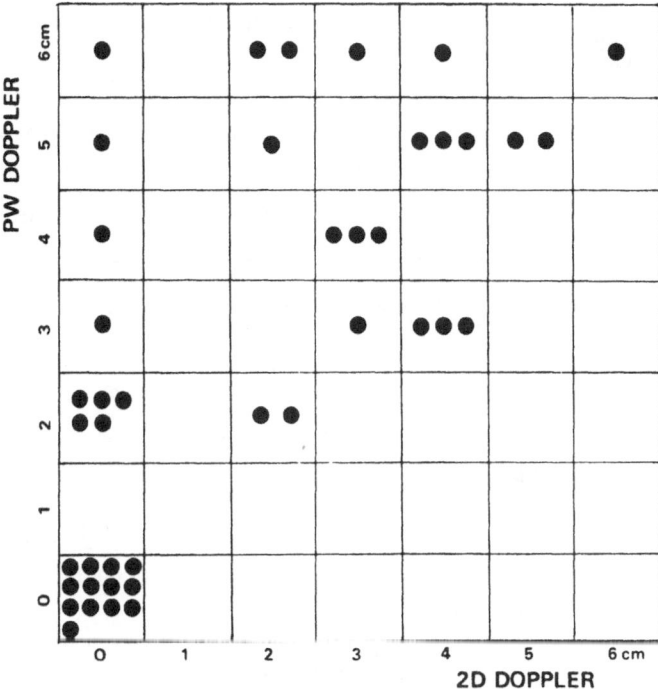

Figure 3. Length of mitral regurgitant jets measured from 2D-Doppler images (abscissa) versus length of jets by pulsed wave mapping using a conventional V-mode pulsed wave instrument (ordinate).

ventricular valves are particularly important with 2D-Doppler, and foreshortening of the conventional echo views to bring the transducer nearer to the atria is a necessary strategy in assessing atrioventricular valvular regurgitation. This is critical in patients with cardiomyopathy in whom a jet of mitral regurgitation, for example, may begin some 8–10 cm from an apical transducer position. Laboratories with long experience in these foreshortening techniques have reported excellent correlation between 2D-Doppler and angiographic grades of severity in regurgitant lesions [7, 8]. For the sake of speed and reliability, however, high priority must still be placed on improving sensitivity of the 2D-Doppler in future generations of equipment.

Prosthetic valves

The considerations discussed above for stenotic and regurgitant native valve lesions apply equally well in the case of prosthetic valve dysfunction. Several unique features of the application of 2D-Doppler to prosthetic valves deserve special consideration.

V-mode Doppler has proven useful in discriminating central from paravalvular

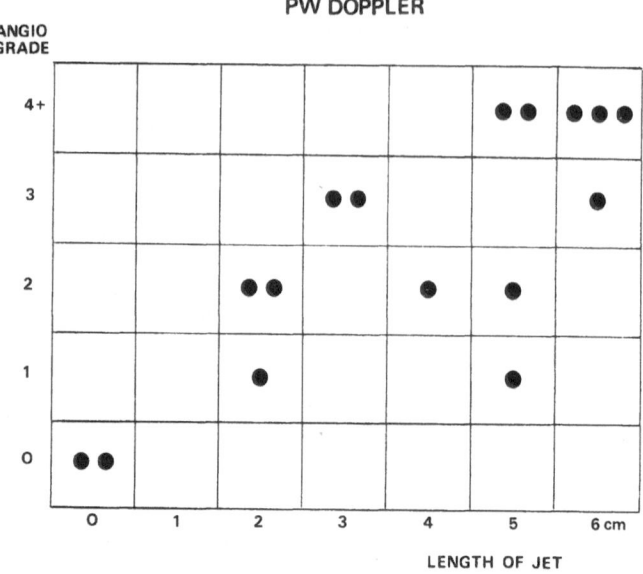

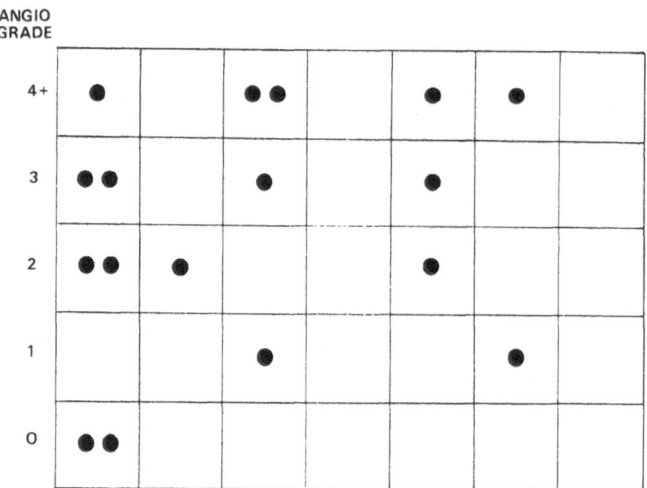

Figure 4. Quantitation of mitral regurgitation by Doppler mapping methods. *Top:* length of jet by pulsed wave Doppler mapping versus angiographic grade of regurgitation. *Bottom:* length of jet by 2D-Doppler mapping versus angiographic grade in the same patient group.

regurgitation in some prosthetic valves. Motion of the heart relative to the Doppler sample volume can make this determination difficult, however, and confident prediction of the site of the regurgitant jet has only been possible in approximately half of the patients we have studied. Two-dimensional Doppler, which provides a direct reference of flow to anatomic structure, may afford more reliable and detailed discrimination of central versus paravalvular leaks in cases where these jets can be recorded well.

There is promising initial work in characterizing the distinctive 2D-Doppler flow patterns of different prosthetic valves [9]. These patterns might potentially provide a 'signature' for a particular valve, to be checked against future studies in the same patient for signs of early degeneration.

An intriguing feature of tissue prosthetic mitral flow, which we and others have noted, is the marked medial deviation of flow (toward the septum) compared to the axis of normal mitral inflow (plate 4). In normals, 2D-Doppler shows mitral inflow directed inferolaterally within the left ventricle, turning medially at the ventricular apex and continuing toward the outflow tract before mechanical systole commences. The usual positioning of porcine prosthetic mitral valves clearly alters this diastolic flow pattern, reversing the direction of normal flow. Inflow begins in a superomedial direction toward the intraventricular septum and then proceeds into the apical region where it turns inferolaterally. This pattern could conceivably represent a significant cost to the ventricle in terms of mechanical efficiency. While such concepts are speculative at present, it is clear that 2D-Doppler can provide a new window on flow dynamics in prosthetic valves, potentially generating information of practical clinical utility.

Ischemic heart disease

Applications of 2D-Doppler technology in patients with coronary disease remain somewhat rudimentary at present. Practical measurement of coronary blood flow is beyond the limits of current transcutaneous Doppler capability. Detection of flow in coronary artery bypass grafts by V-mode Doppler has been reported but is technically difficult. Two-dimensional Doppler has not been systematically applied to this problem. Although 2D-Doppler analysis of segmental wall motion velocity has been suggested as a theoretically attractive measure of regional wall mechanics, this also remains in the speculative realm. Two-dimensional Doppler should be useful in assessing changes in intracavitary left ventricular blood flow caused by aneurysms and might provide new insight into the *in vivo* properties of flow which contribute to thrombus formation. At present there is no published experience in this area. Post-infarction ventricular septal defect, pseudo-aneurysm and contained acute cardiac rupture are complications of ischemic heart disease which may be more easily recognized by the 2D-Doppler method compared to conventional 2D imaging alone.

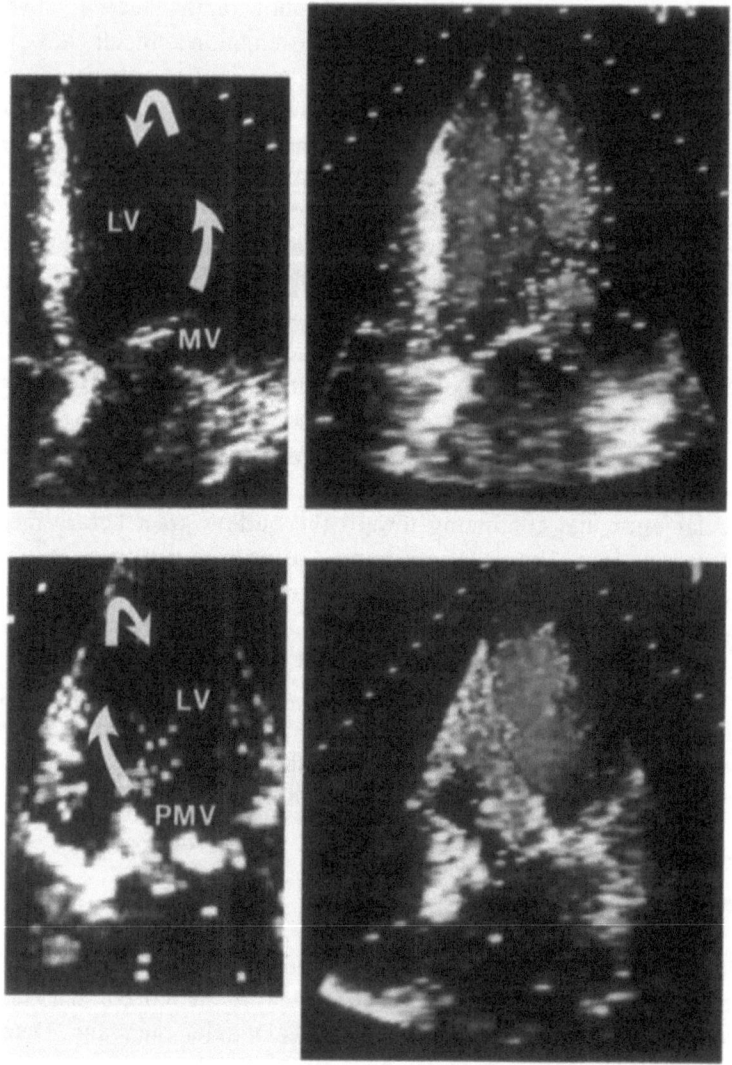

Plate 4. Top: mitral inflow, native valve (Aloka). Flow through the mitral valve (MV) is directed inferolaterally into the ventricle (orange), then turns medially at the apex and continues into the left ventricular outflow tract (blue). LV = left ventricle. *Bottom:* mitral inflow, Hancock tissue prosthesis (Aloka). Flow is initially directed superomedially (orange), continues along the interventricular septum to the apex, and then turns laterally (blue). PMV = prosthetic mitral valve; LV = left ventricle.

Cardiac output

Current techniques of Doppler-based cardiac output determination suffer from two major limitations: (a) it is essential to determine a cross-sectional area representing the boundaries of flow at the site being sampled (e.g., the aortic cross-sectional area); and (b) it is necessary to assume that the flow profile at the site is effectively flat (i.e., all of the blood cells at that site are moving at one, uniform velocity). In theory, 2D-Doppler can help eliminate both of these limitations.

In a preliminary report of cardiac output studies on dogs, Hoit *et al.* [10] found that cross-sectional flow areas determined by 2D-Doppler were significantly smaller (0.70–0.73x) than the corresponding anatomic areas at all four valve sites. The measured 2D-Doppler flow areas correlated well with the calculated flow areas based on measured cardiac output and V-mode Doppler flow integrals. Data from the same group indicated that cardiac output determinations using the flow diameter measured from the 2D-Doppler image gave more accurate results than the use of an anatomic (2D echo) dimension at low cardiac outputs (where the flow profile may be parabolic rather than flat) [11]. Theoretically, inhomogeneity of flow profiles due to a variety of conditions could be directly visualized by 2D-Doppler and hence this technique could be used to screen patients to assess suitability for Doppler output determinations.

Conclusions and overview

The unique advantage of 2D-Doppler over other noninvasive techniques is that it displays a geographic map of flow velocities which is referenced precisely to anatomic structures. The power of this new technology in application to complex congenital heart disease is becoming increasingly clear. In adult cardiology, where coronary and valvular heart disease account for the bulk of diagnostic efforts, established applications of the 2D-Doppler technology are more limited. This discussion has reviewed the potential usefulness of 2D-Doppler in improving the quantitative Doppler estimation of transvalvular pressure gradients, in providing semiquantitative assessment of regurgitant lesions, in providing special information both in the evaluation of prosthetic heart valves and on the effects of coronary disease on ventricular function and in improving the accuracy of Doppler-based cardiac output determinations.

Although the focus of the studies reviewed here has been on quantitative applications of 2D-Doppler, it is worth emphasizing that the unique qualitative display capability of the device can be extremely useful in its own right by providing orientation to the operator performing a cardiac ultrasound examination. An initial scan of the heart in the 2D-Doppler mode may be used to quickly determine areas of easily imaged valvular or shunt pathology and thereby help the operator to organize the complete ultrasound examination. Use of the 2D-Doppler mode for orientation of the pulsed or continuous wave beam may significantly streamline the examination of both stenotic and regurgitant valvular lesions.

It is in this context of improved overall efficiency that the usefulness of 2D-Doppler for adult cardiology will ultimately be decided. At the present stage of development, 2D-Doppler adds a limited amount of information to the conventional echo/Doppler examination in adults. The practical issue is whether a given laboratory will find the addition of 2D-Doppler capability to be worth the extra cost by providing a more streamlined and reliable Doppler study than is possible with current equipment.

References

1. Hatle L, Angelsen B: Doppler Ultrasound in Cardiology, pp. 124–143. Philadelphia: Lea and Febiger, 1985.
2. Nakagawa H, Miyatake K, Izumi S, Kinoshita N, Sakakibara H, Nimura Y: Application of real-time two-dimensional Doppler flow imaging system for the measurement of pressure gradient across the mitral valve in mitral stenosis. J Am Coll Cardiol 5: 403 (Abstract), 1985.
3. Abbasi A, Allen M, DeCristofaro D, Ungar I: Detection and estimation of the degree of mitral regurgitation by range-gated pulsed Doppler echocardiography. Circulation 61: 143–147, 1980.
4. Veyrat C, Ameur A, Bas S, Lessana A, Abitbol G, Kalmanson D: Pulsed Doppler echocardiographic indices to for assessing mitral regurgitation. Br Heart J 51: 130–138, 1984.
5. Miyatake K, Kinoshita N, Nagata S, Beppu S, Park Y, Sakakibara H, Nimura Y: Intracardiac flow pattern in mitral regurgitation studied with combined use of ultrasonic pulsed Doppler techniques and cross-sectional echocardiography. Am J Cardiol 45: 155–162, 1980.
6. Yock P, Segal J, Teirstein P, Schnittger I, Popp R: Doppler color flow mapping: utility in valvular regurgitation. Circulation 70 (Suppl II): II–38 (Abstract), 1984.
7. Omoto R, Yokote Y, Takamoto S, Kyo S, Ueda K, Asano H, Namekawa K, Kasai C, Kondo Y, Koyano A: The development of real-time two-dimensional Doppler echocardiography and its clinical significance in acquired valvular heart diseases. Jpn Heart J 25: 325–340, 1984.
8. Kitabatake A, Masuyama T, Asao M, Tanouchi J, Morita T, Ito H, Hori M, Inoug M, Abe H: Noninvasive estimation of the degree of regurgitation from two-dimensional (2-D) Doppler-Echo (flow structure) cardiac image. Circulation 69 (Suppl III): III–367 (Abstract), 1983.
9. Bommer W, Tam K, Ehret R, Rebeck K: 2-D real-time flow mapping of prosthetic heart valves. J Am Coll Cardiol 5: 526 (Abstract), 1985.
10. Hoit B, Bhargava V, Swensson R, Sattn D: Determination of flow area in echo Doppler calculations of cardiac output: investigations of flow orifices using real-time, two-dimensional echo Doppler color flow mapping. Circulation 70 (Suppl II): II–39 (Abstract), 1984.
11. Valdes-Cruz L, Elias W, Dalton N, Hagan-Ansert S, Sahn D, Swensson R, Sherman F: Comparison of cardiac flows calculated with color coded Doppler flow mapping and conventional Doppler techniques: validation studies in an open chest animal model. J Am Coll Cardiol 5: 452 (Abstract), 1985.

Color flow imaging and conventional two-dimensional pulsed Doppler echocardiography: selected observations and experience

J. Geoffrey Stevenson

In 1978, Brandestini and co-workers at the University of Washington produced a 128 channel digital multigate Doppler instrument [1, 2] which, for the first time in clinical ultrasound, allowed imaging of cardiac structure and blood flow in real time. Clinical trials suggested utility in evaluation of a variety of defects, including atrial and ventricular septal defects, patent ductus arteriosus, and atrioventricular valve regurgitation [3–5]. That multigate Doppler device was introduced into a Doppler field at a time when the credibility and acceptance of Doppler techniques had not yet occurred in many areas. While the color Doppler format was greeted with interest, it was considered by many to be just an interesting 'gimick'. American journals felt that the instrument, and reports of its utility to be too preliminary to deserve priority sufficient to publish. Reports of the initial applications thus appeared in the more open minded European literature. The Brandestini instrument remained a uniquely curious unit, and did not progress toward commercial availability. At about the same time, our Japanese colleagues were engaged in work toward production of a commercially available real time flow imaging system. Because of barriers imposed by language and communication, neither center was fully aware of each other's activity. But, with the introduction of the Japanese system, at a later time when Doppler techniques had come to be accepted, an enthusiastic resurgence in interest in color flow imaging was noted.[6].

The purpose of this communication is to summarize some of the applications of flow imaging which have evolved within our experience since 1978. These observations are by necessity highly selected. I have chosen to include only patients who were examined with at least one color flow device, and one conventional two-dimensional Doppler device at the same setting, which was usually at catheterization. In many of the cases, it was impossible to blind the examiner to the results of the other Doppler modality.

The conventional Doppler instrumentation evolved and varied over the time period, and included the original 1976 UW Duplex scanner. Most of the examinations were performed with time-current ATL instruments. Most of the color flow examinations were performed with the Brandestini multigate Doppler, a small number with the Aloka device [6], and a few with a variety of other prototype color flow imaging systems. Common to all the color flow systems is display of solid structure in white color, with directional blood flow display in other colors. The Brandestini instrument is used almost exclusively in M-mode format because of a lower than desirable two dimensional frame rate for pediatrics. Though the frame rate for the Aloka system is also low, it can be used in either two dimensional, or M-mode format. It should be noted that the colors chosen for directional flow display by Brandestini and colleagues in 1978 differ from those employed in the Aloka instrument. Flow toward the transducer is blue/green in the Brandestini unit, but orange/red with the Aloka. Flow away from the transducer is red/orange in the Brandestini unit, and blue with the Aloka. Additionally, turbulence is displayed as an addition of turquoise color with the Aloka system, while the Brandestini device displays turbulence based on characteristic mixture of directions and velocities. These differences must be kept in mind in review of the figures in this chapter.

For ventricular septal defect, we look for flow within the ventricular septum, either by conventional two dimensional Doppler (Figure 1), or by color flow (Figure 2) [7–9]. As most ventricular shunts are oriented favorably for detection from precordial or subcostal approaches, little difficulty has been encountered in their detection. One must be careful however to clearly demonstrate flow through the septum; right ventricular turbulence by conventional Doppler does not prove ventricular septal defect [7], while with color flow, confusion of tricuspid inflow could lead to a false positive diagnosis if one is careless and fails to clearly demonstrate the origin of a flow signal. Experience from two periods is shown in Table 1. Sensitivity and specificity are high for both conventional Doppler and color flow. For practical purposes, ventricular septal defect can be detected with either Doppler technique, with equal accuracy.

Direction of ventricular septal defect flow has important clinical implications [9]. Examples of left to right ventricular shunting are shown in Figures 2 and 3, and right to left ventricular shunting in Figures 4 and 5. Experience with direction of shunting is summarized in Table 2. It is noted that direction of flow as determined by conventional Doppler agreed fairly well with catheterization ($r = 0.89$). With color flow however, the correspondence with catheterization was considerably better ($r = 0.99$). The explanation for this may be that with conventional Doppler, flow is sampled at a fixed point in the heart, and that with cardiac motion the stationary sample volume may actually be on different sides of the defect at different times. With color flow systems, flow is displayed upon structure throughout the motion of the cardiac cycle, and hence directional information, as displayed upon structure, should be more accurate.

The location and number of ventricular septal defects is clinically important. An example of a large muscular defect is shown in Figure 3. In Figure 5, is shown an apical defect in color flow format of the Brandestini unit. The same patient's

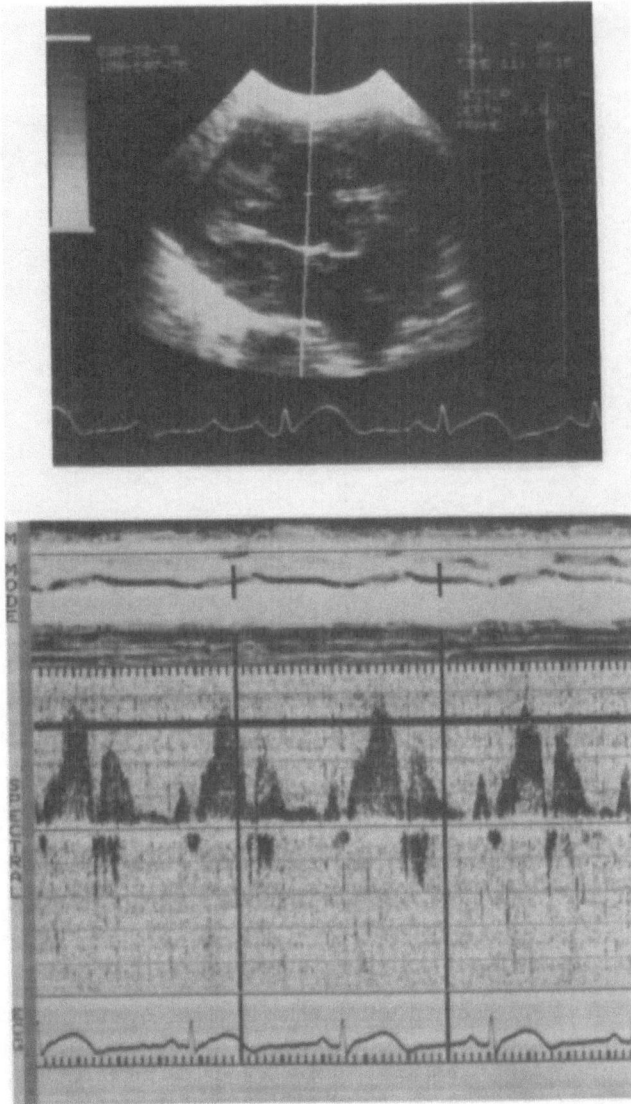

Figure 1. Ventricular septal defect, conventional two-dimensional Doppler. From parasternal long axis approach, the Doppler sample volume (white dot) has been placed in a large ventricular septal defect (VSD). The right and left ventricles (RV, LV) are shown, along with aorta (AO) and left atrium (LA). On the Doppler flow record, the compressed M-mode at the top shows the solid line position of the sample volume within the VSD. From a central zero line, spectral broadening is evident, with upward Doppler shift; turbulent left to right VSD flow.

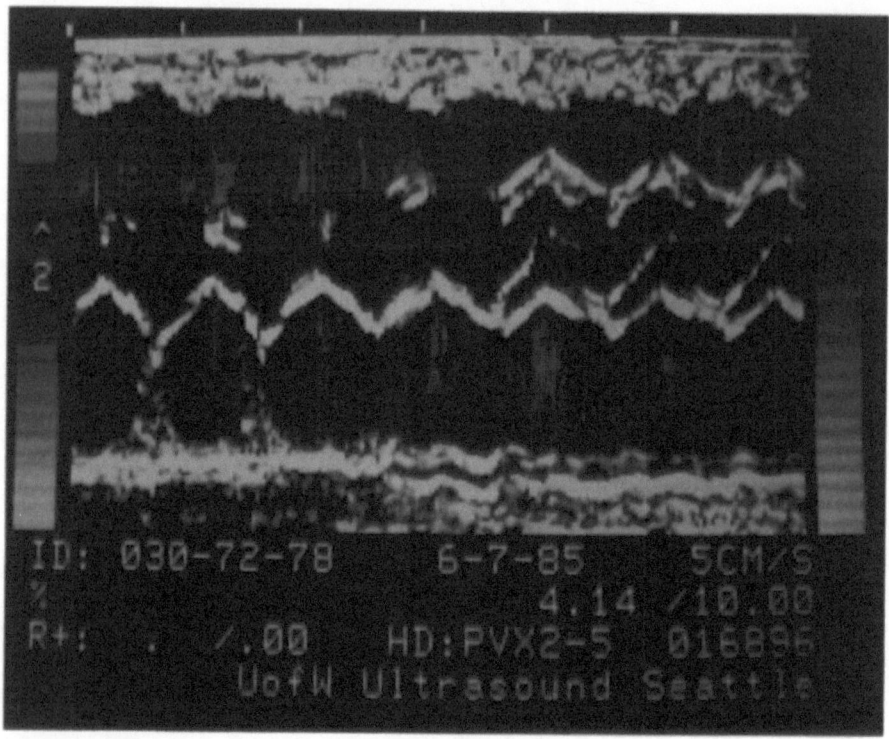

Figure 2. Multigate Doppler recording of VSD flow. The same patient shown in Figure 1 is examined with the Brandestini Doppler. Solid structures are shown in white, in M-mode format. The aortic root appears toward the right, and on the left of the figure, a sweep to the ventricles is shown. The white septal echo drops out and is replaced by blue green directional colors. As blue green colors indicate flow toward the transducer, this VSD shunt is left to right.

right to left apical shunt is also shown in Figure 6 using a conventional ATL Doppler system. As seen in Table 3, color flow led to better detection of apical defects, but was no more accurate than conventional Doppler for detection of defects at other levels. While conventional Doppler performed about as well as catheterization in demonstration of multiple defects, color flow proved considerably more accurate (Table 4). The reason for improved accuracy with color flow stems from the ease of recognition of visualized flow. The failures with conventional Doppler stem from failure to place the sample volume in the correct location for diagnosis. Color flow displays cover many portions of the heart at one time and obviate the need for sequential single sample volume placement.

Doppler detection of patent ductus arteriosus depends upon demonstration of flow through the ductus into the pulmonary artery [10–12]. A conventional Doppler example is shown in Figure 7. Using the Brandestini system (Figures 8 and 9), the directional ductal flow into the pulmonary artery is readily evident. Over the years our highest diagnostic accuracy for conventional Doppler has been

Table 1. Ventricular septal defect.

	Cath/angio		Sensitivity	Specificity
	+	−		
1981:				
2D/Doppler			96%	99%
+	227	2		
−	9	240		
Color flow			98%	100%
+	140	0		
−	3	94		
1984:				
2D/Doppler			96%	99%
+	369	3		
−	13	591		
Color flow			98%	99%
+	316	1		
−	6	298		

with patent ductus. As can be seen in Table 5, color flow has not led to an improvement in accuracy. But with patent ductus and a number of other lesions, color flow has provided clues as to common locations of disturbed flow. The sample volume placement shown in Figure 7, along the anterior wall of the pulmonary artery, has been advocated for years as a 'good' location for detection of patent ductus flow. Using the same orientation, Figure 10 shows that the turbulent jet of the ductus indeed courses long the anterior wall of the pulmonary artery, as if adherent to it. This natural flow pattern of patent ductus is vividly shown in color flow format, having only been inferred from conventional Doppler experience.

Many centers have reported high accuracy for conventional Doppler in evaluation of atrioventricular valve regurgitation in adults and children; the experience has been summarized recently [12]. We have reported early experience with color flow imaging in detection and assessment of severity based upon demonstration of the breadth and extent of regurgitant flow [5]. Using conventional two dimensional Doppler, sample volume placement at the valve, and posterior to it, may allow detection of systolic spectral broadening. The breadth and extent of the jet may be assessed by careful sequential sample volume positioning throughout the atrium. Color flow systems may also be used to display regurgitant flow as shown in Figure 11 and Figure 12 with the Aloka and Brandestini systems on the same patient.

As shown in Table 6, both conventional Doppler and color flow have equal accuracy for detection of regurgitation in our series. Others have noted slightly

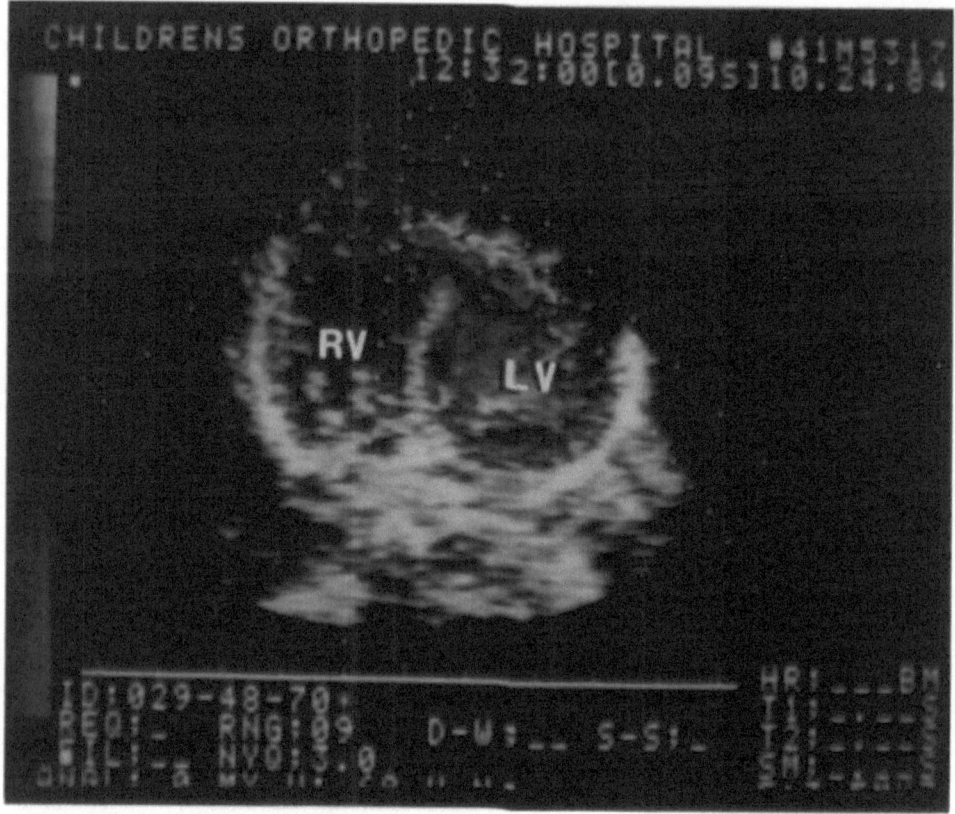

Figure 3. Left to right ventricular septal defect, two-dimensional color flow. From parasternal short axis approach, the right and left ventricles (RV, LV) have been imaged. An orange jet through the ventricular septum, in low position, is readily apparent. In the Aloka system, orange colors indicate flow toward the transducer, so this is a left to right VSD shunt.

lesser sensitivity for detection with the Aloka device in adult patients [14–15]. The better sensitivity with the Brandestini instrument probably stems from its capability for display of lower regurgitant velocities which may go undisplayed, undetected, on the Aloka system.

Using previously described criteria for assessment of severity in infants and small children [5] we have noted good correlation with ventriculography when regurgitation has been assessed by conventional Doppler (r = 0.89). However when the Brandestini instrument has been used for color flow assessment of severity, the correlation with ventriculography has been excellent (r = 0.98) (Table 7). The likely explanation for the superiority of color flow imaging in this application is similar to that postulated for improved results with direction of ventricular septal defect flow: color flow depiction of structure and flow together throughout time is more accurate than depiction of flow at a fixed point through or about which cardiac structures move.

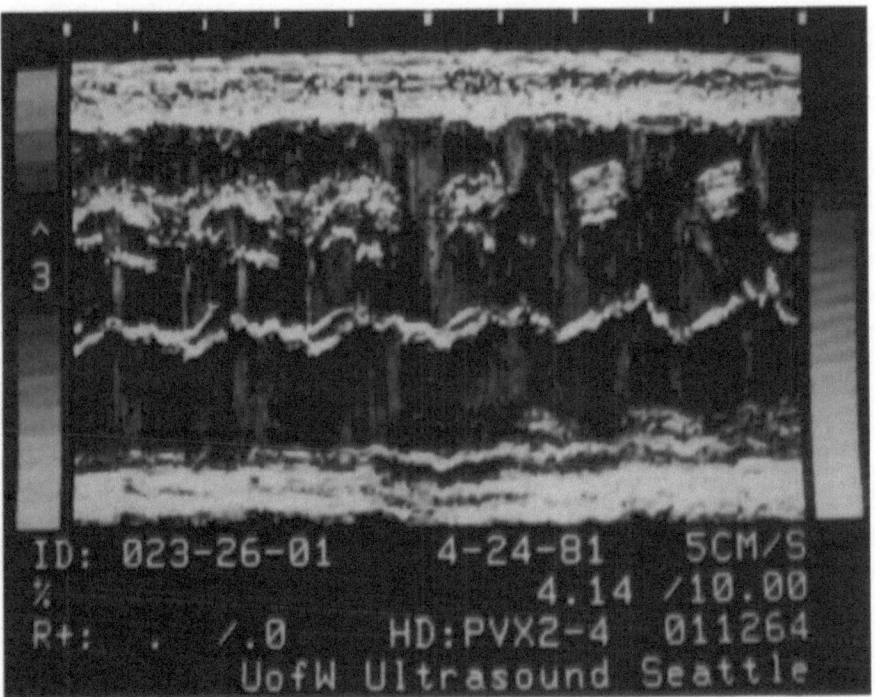

Figure 4. Multigate Doppler recording of right to left VSD flow. The approach and orientation is similar to that shown in Figure 2. The white septal echo is replaced by orange colors indicating flow away from the transducer on the Brandestini system, or a right to left VSD shunt.

There have been reports of difficulty in detecting mild, low velocity mitral regurgitation with the Aloka system. Difficulty arises when non angle corrected velocities fall below the threshold for color display. We have felt that this may also lead to difficulties in tracking the breadth and extent of regurgitant flow. In Figure 11 a blue jet of regurgitation is evident. It would seem to extend only a small distance from the valve, and the remainder of the atrium is black. With single sample volume placement at the edge of the blue jet, (Figure 11–1), and further into the atrium, regurgitant flow is clearly detected by conventional Doppler, well into the regions of the atrium which appear black (no-regurgitation) in Figure 11–2. The same patient, examined on the Brandestini instrument (Figure 12), could clearly be shown to have a relatively low velocity jet of regurgitation which extended several centimeters to the atrial wall. In a small comparison series (Table 8), we encountered difficulty in accurately estimating the severity of regurgitation with the Aloka system. Based on that experience which is not unique to our hospital, it seem wise to also evaluate color flow-detected regurgitant jets with conventional Doppler, in terms of breadth and extent of the regurgitant jets.

Demonstration of flow through the atrial septum has been the diagnositic

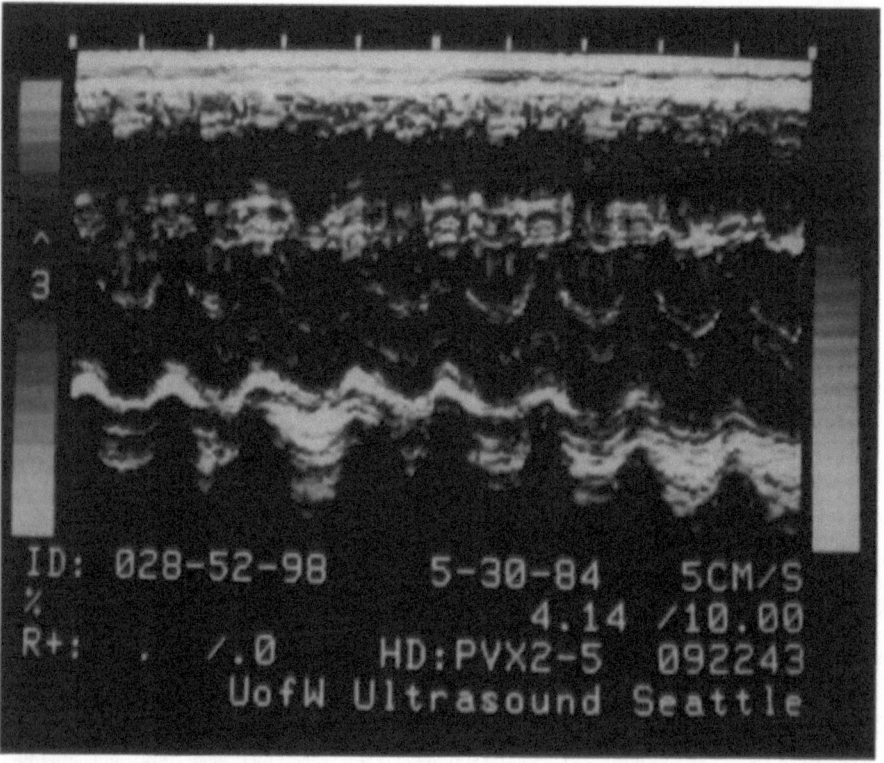

Figure 5. Apical ventricular septal defect, multigate Doppler, right to left shunt. From precordial approach, a section is obtained similar to the 2D format shown in the following figure from the same patient. The apical portion of the ventricular septum is shown in white, with orange color replacement of the low apical portion of the septum, indicating right to left VSD flow in this location. See Figure 6.

criterion for invasive and noninvasive diagnosis [7, 16]. Accuracy for conventional Doppler has been high for detection [16] and location of atrial defects. In our experience, no further increase in accuracy has come from color flow imaging. This is probably because the atrial septum is not a difficult structure to evaluate with conventional Doppler. Color flow evaluation of the atrial septum however can be useful in demonstrating the origin of disturbed flow, and associated defects. Figure 15 shows color through a primum defect, clearly in a location quite different from the post-septostomy atrial shunt shown in Figure 16. While these defects are readily detectable on two dimensional echo alone, the color flow dramatically calls attention to their presence. In patients with primum defects, mitral regurgitation may be commonly encountered. The patient in Figure 13 has no apparent regurgitation, while Figure 15 in another patient clearly shows a rather extensive regurgitant blue jet. As its direction and location differ from the shunt flow, there is no confusion between the two flow disturbances in the left atrium.

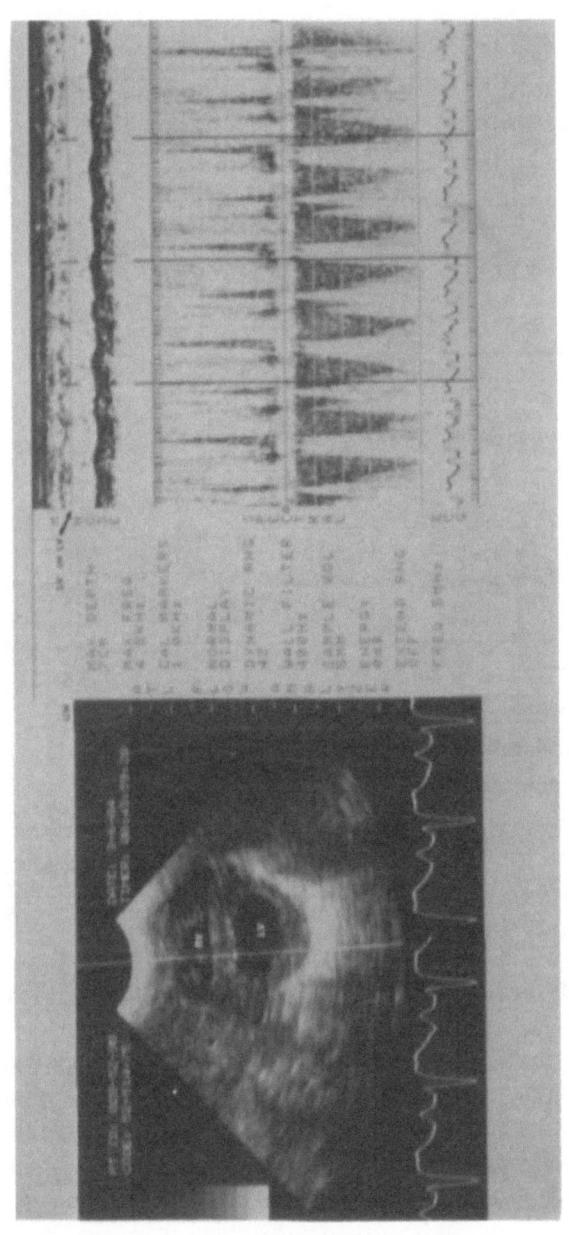

Figure 6. Conventional Doppler demonstration of apical VSD. This is the same patient shown in Figure 5, examined on different days, but under similar conditions. In short axis 2D orientation, the right and left ventricles (RV, LV) are shown, with sample volume placement on the LV side of the lower portion of the septum. From that location, right to left (downward deflection) VSD flow is recorded.

Table 2. Direction of ventricular septal defect flow.

	Invasive study			r
	L-R	BD	R-L	
2D/Doppler				0.89
L-R	51	2		
BD	9	17	4	
R-L			17	
Color flow				0.99
L-R	54	2		
BD	6	17		
R-L			21	

Table 3. Location of ventricular septal defect.

	Color	2D/Doppler	Surgeon
High	140 (98%)	142 (99%)	143
Inflow	15 (94%)*	15 (94%)	16
Apical/Muscular	26 (100%)*	83 (88%)	26

* One false positive each

Table 4. Multiple ventricular septal defect.

Cath/angio	21/28	79%
2D/Doppler	21/28	75%
Color flow	26/28	93%

Color flow has fascinated many with its vivid delineation of the characteristics of various flow disturbances. From our early presentations of conventional Doppler records in atrial septal defect [7], question was commonly raised as to the origin, significance and reality of the disturbed flow on the left atrial side of left to right shunting atrial defects. Most had expected the flow disturbance to appear only downstream from the defect, in the right atrium. Inspection of Figures 13–15 clearly shows that the disturbed velocities are indeed present on the left atrial side of these defects.

The magnitude of atrial shunts is commonly estimated from the degree of right heart enlargement on M-mode and two dimensional echo. The breadth and extent of the disturbed velocities arising through atrial defects has also been proposed as in estimator of shunt size [17]. The use of chamber dimensions to

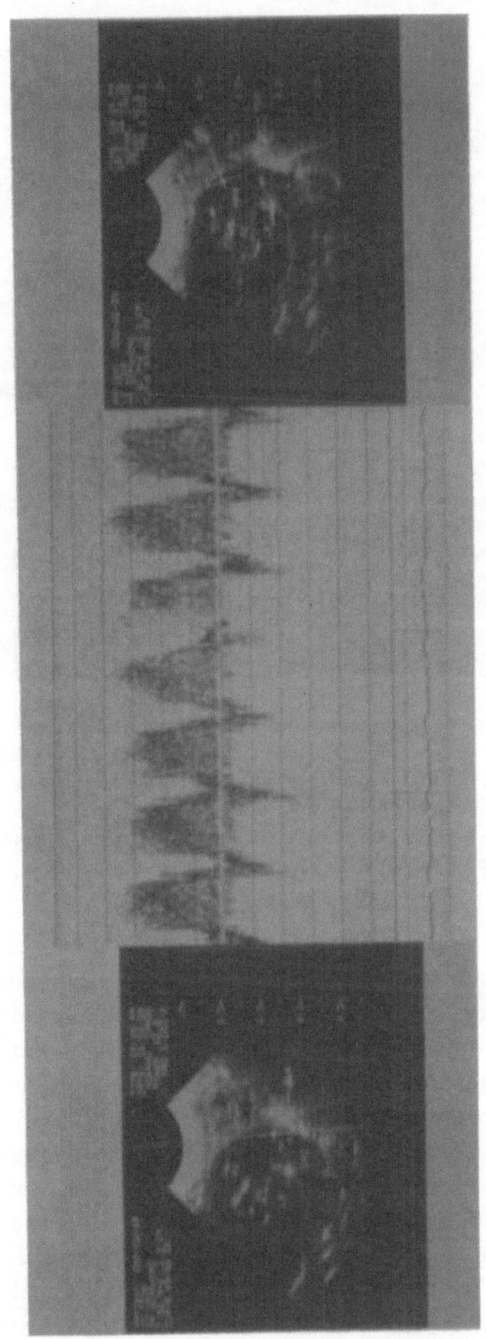

Figure 7. Two-dimensional Doppler diagnosis of patent ductus arteriosus. On the left, the Doppler sample volume has been placed in the ductus itself, and on the right, the sample volume is positioned along the anterior aspect of the main pulmonary artery. A flow recording from that latter position demonstrates pandiastolic turbulence directed into the pulmonary artery, in left to right direction. (PV = pulmonary valve, AO = aorta, LA = left atrium, DAO = descending thoracic aorta, PDA = patent ductus arteriosus).

94

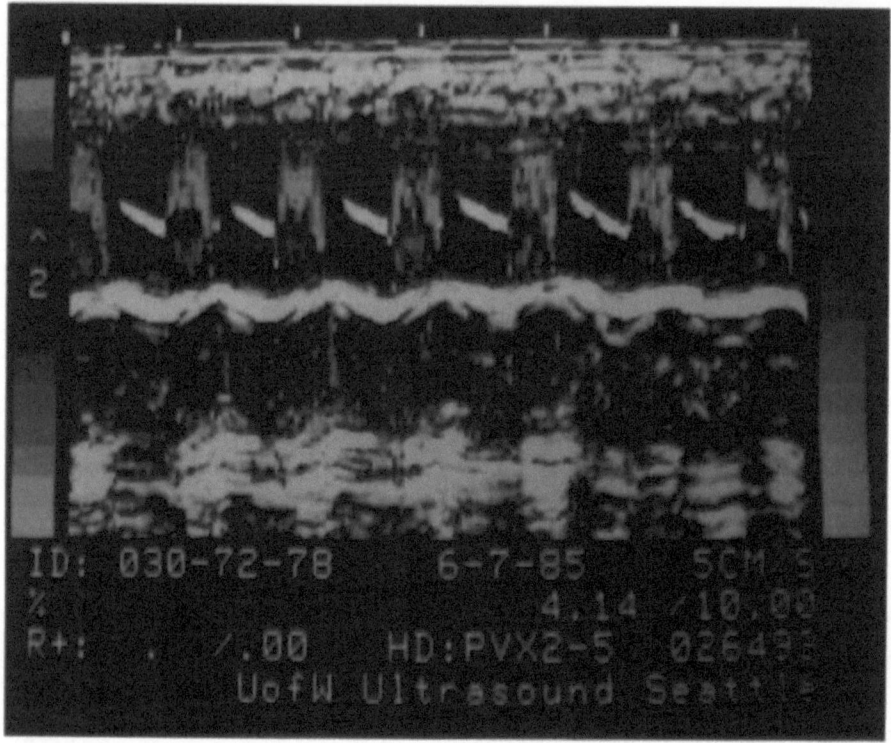

Figure 8. Multigate Doppler, normal pulmonary valve and pulmonary artery flow. From a precordial approach similar to Figure 7, right, the normal pulmonary valve appears in white. During systole, there is orange color flow indicating normal flow away from the transducer into the pulmonary artery. As peak systolic velocity exceeds the set limits for color display at the time of this recording, the center of the systolic flow appears in green indicative of aliasing (wrap-around to the opposite directional color). Note that distal to the pulmonary valve in diastole there is no directional color flow, and thus the record is black.

estimate shunt size assumes that all of a given chamber dilitation is due to the shunt; additional lesions are presumed to be absent. Color flow detection or exclusion of tricuspid regurgitation in patients with atrial defects could be employed for more accurate interpretation of right heart enlargement.

From the experience abstracted and summarized here, color flow imaging has led to improvements in detection of disturbed flow in only a few situations. But, these have been important contributions as they have improved our overall noninvasive diagnosis. Color flow has proven superior in assessment of regurgitation, providing one is careful and cognizant of limitations; at times, conventional Doppler is needed for definition. Color flow has the unique capability for spatial display of flow characteristics. These are important contributions of new technology; one should not have expected color flow to dramatically surpass the already formidable capabilities of conventional two dimensional Doppler!

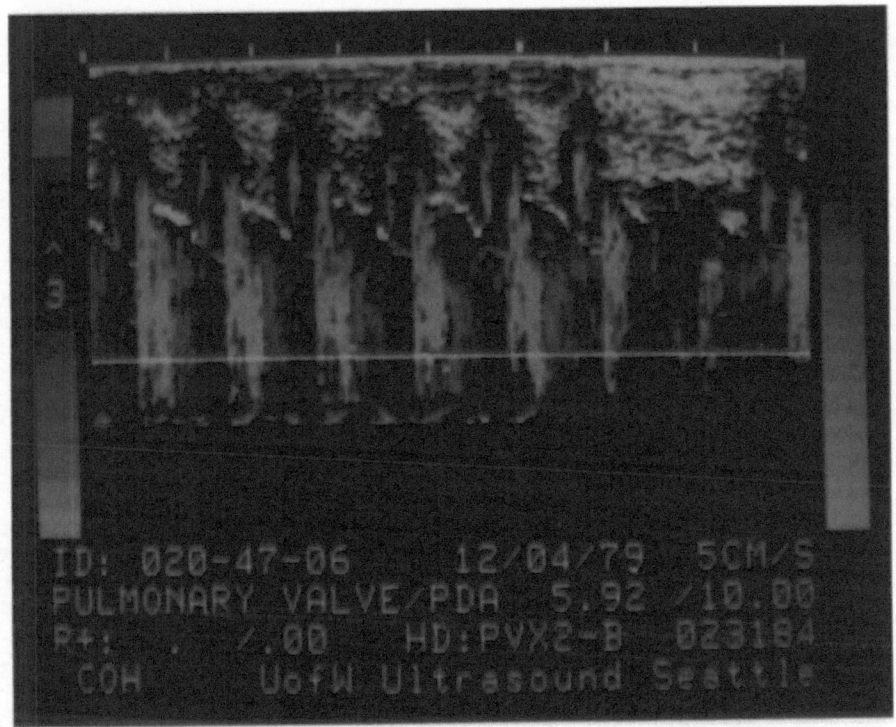

Figure 9. Multigate Doppler, patent ductus arteriosus. Orientation is similar to that shown in Figure 8. Yellow/orange systolic flow is normal. But during diastole, there is blue green color distal to the pulmonary valve, indicating flow toward the transducer from the patent ductus. Compare with Figure 7, center.

Table 5. Patent ductus arteriosus.

	Cath/angio/surgery		Sensitivity	Specificity
	+	−		
2D/Doppler			99%	100%
+	612	0		
−	6	591		
Color flow			99%	100%
+	199	0		
−	3	201		

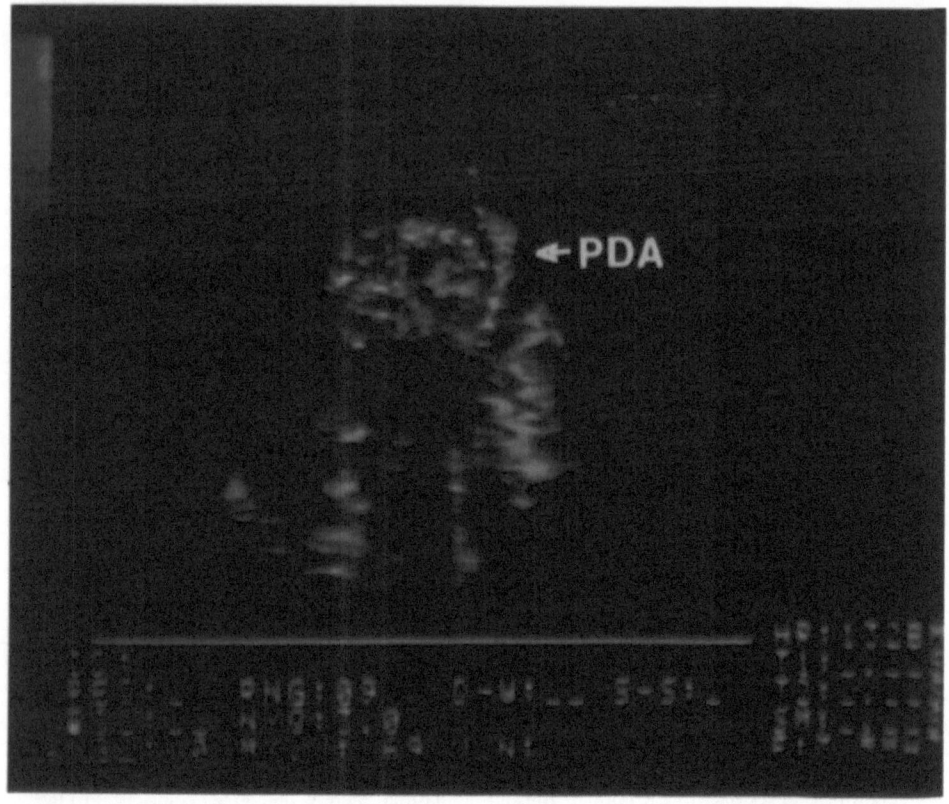

Figure 10. Two-dimensional color flow, patent ductus arteriosus. The orientation and approach is similar to that shown in Figure 7. The flow from the descending aorta into the pulmonary artery appears as a yellow jet with turquoise mixture along the edges, and is labeled as PDA. The flow courses along the anterior aspect of the main pulmonary artery, similar to Figure 7. Examination performed by the author at Saitama Medical School, Saitama, Japan, courtesy of Dr. Ryozo Omoto.

In considering the actual and potential advantages over conventional Doppler, it is likely that the impact of each of these will vary from center to center, depending upon individual experience with Doppler. In our hands, color flow has clearly led to quicker detection of flow disturbances in many cases, obviating the time-consuming careful and methodical sample volume placements required with conventional Doppler. Color flow has proven useful in screening for flow disturbances, and in detection of quite unexpected flow disturbances. As more and more is being asked from a cardiac ultrasound evaluation, there is a great need to quickly identify areas of abnormality. Consider for example the time and care required to differentiate and evaluate disturbed left ventricular outflow tract flow. With conventional Doppler, excellent technique is required to differentiate aortic regurgitation jets from mitral stenosis jets; they appear remarkably similar on conventional Doppler (Figure 16). but in color format, Figure 17, the number

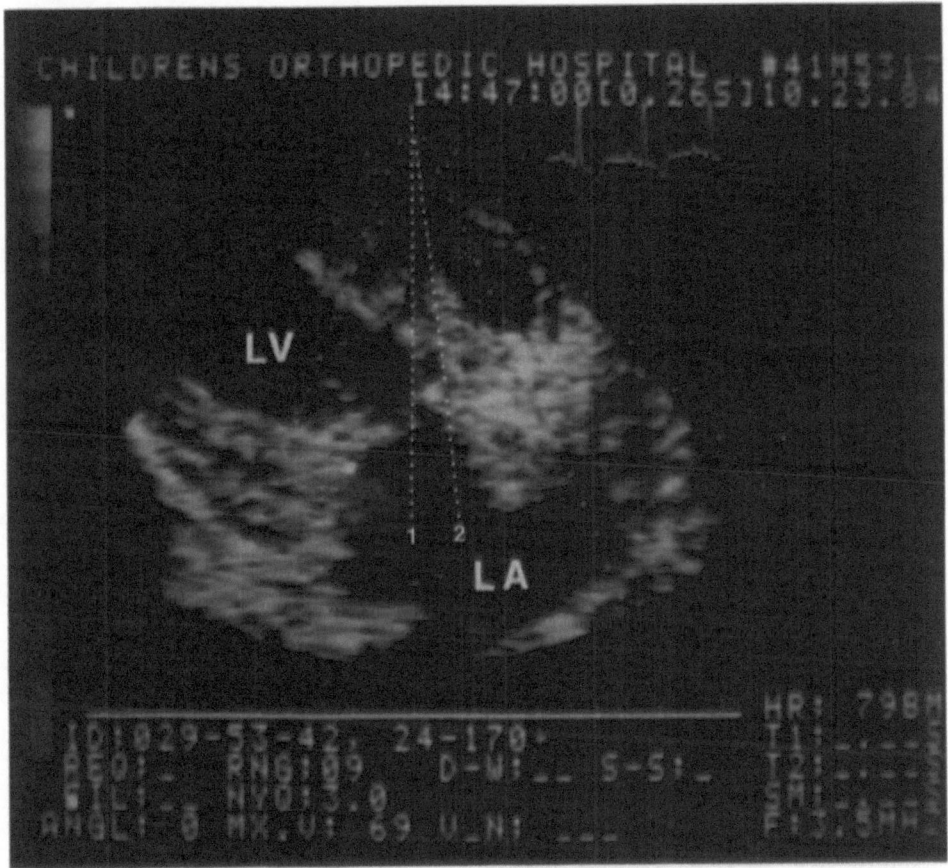

Figure 11. Two-dimensional color flow mitral regurgitation. In two dimensional format, the left ventricle and left atrium (LV, LA) are imaged. A blue jet of mitral regurgitation is seen to extend posterior to the mitral valve, in a patient with endocardial cushion defect. Conventional sample volume placement at the edge of the blue jet is shown by position #1, and placement in the left atrium distant from the margin of the imaged jet is indicated by position #2, see text for discussion.

and spatial distribution of the jets is readily evident. Once detected and defined by color flow, one can chose the best Doppler modality for further quantitative assessment. We have also noted a remarkable benefit of color flow in terms of communication. Its nearly angiographic format makes it relatively easy for one to quickly show location, breadth and extent of disturbed flows. Acceptance of noninvasive diagnosis by our surgical colleagues can only be expected to increase through the depiction of structure and flow together.

The limitations of color flow imaging relate to its young age, cost and availability. Currently available instrumentation, however dramatic and impressive [6, 18] will evolve with time, just as has been seen with conventional Doppler systems. It is perhaps unfair to compare prototype color units, or early production

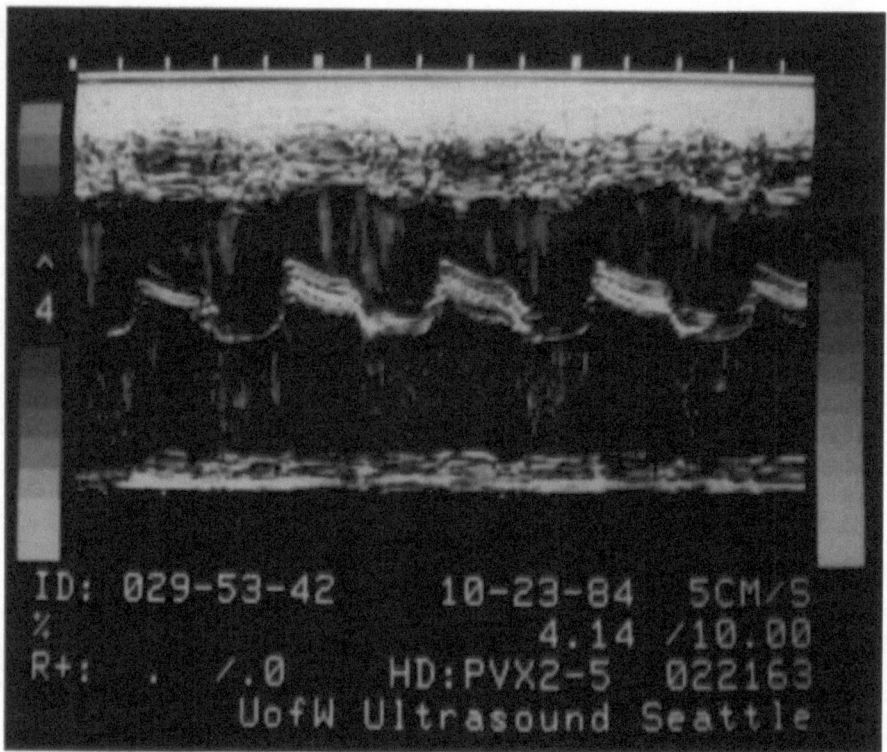

ID: 029-53-42   10-23-84   5CM/S
%   4.14 /10.00
R+:   . /.0   HD:PVX2-5   022163
            UofW Ultrasound Seattle

Figure 12. Multigate Doppler, mitral regurgitation. Using the Brandestini instrument, the same patient shown in Figure 12 has been examined at the same setting. From an apical approach, the mitral valve appears in white. Posterior to the valve in systole, orange and red colors indicate regurgitation, with the color jet extending 3 cm to the atrial wall.

units with refined conventional Doppler systems. However unfair, it is quite interesting to see just how very well the new technological advancements have fared; a tribute to the capabilities of these systems! Currently available color flow intruments are decidedly expensive, and while strong in color flow imaging of course, they are less capable for performance of the remaining aspects of a cardiac ultrasound examination; improvements are to be expected.

Unambiguous display of flow velocities can be a problem with conventional as well as color flow Doppler systems. With conventional Doppler, high velocities have been the primary difficulty; with color flow, there are problems with display of high velocities (Figures 8, 17), as well as failure to display low velocities (Figure 11). One needs to be aware of these problems, be able to recognize their manifestations in individual examinations, and have the instrument and technical flexibility to resolve them.

However enthusiastic we have been about the logical display of structure and flow together, the impact of that display in real time is quite overwhelming. One

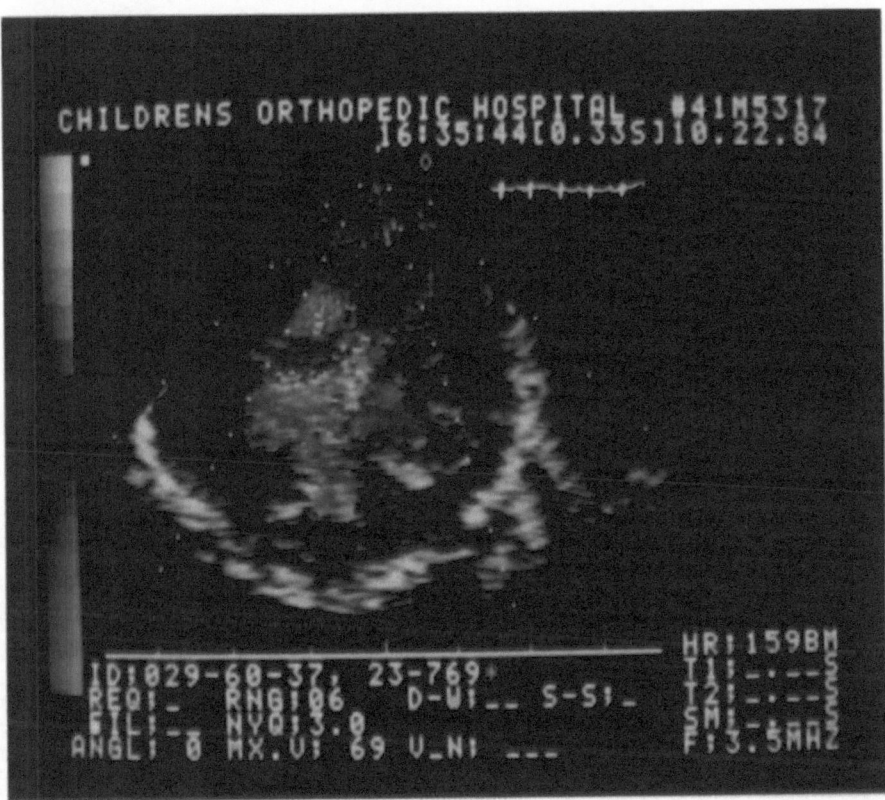

Figure 13. Two-dimensional color flow, ostium primum atrial septal defect. From conventional subcostal four chamber approach, the atria and ventricles have been imaged in white. There is a broad orange jet beginning in the left atrium, and extending through the lower portion of the atrial septum indicating left to right primum ASD flow. Posterior to the mitral valve in systole, there is no reversal of flow colors, no regurgitation. Compare with Figure 15.

Table 6. Atrioventricular valve regurgiation.

	Ventriculography		Sensitivity	Specificity
	+	−		
2D/Doppler:			96%	98%
+	155	4		
−	7	163		
Color flow:			96%	98%
+	94	2		
−	4	99		

Table 7. Atrioventricular valve regurgitation: breadth and extent.

	Ventriculography			r
	Mild	Moderate	Severe	
2D/Doppler				0.89
Mild	156	12	2	
Moderate	12	84	6	
Severe		1	56	
Color flow				0.98
Mild	82	2		
Moderate	4	61	7	
Severe		1	42	

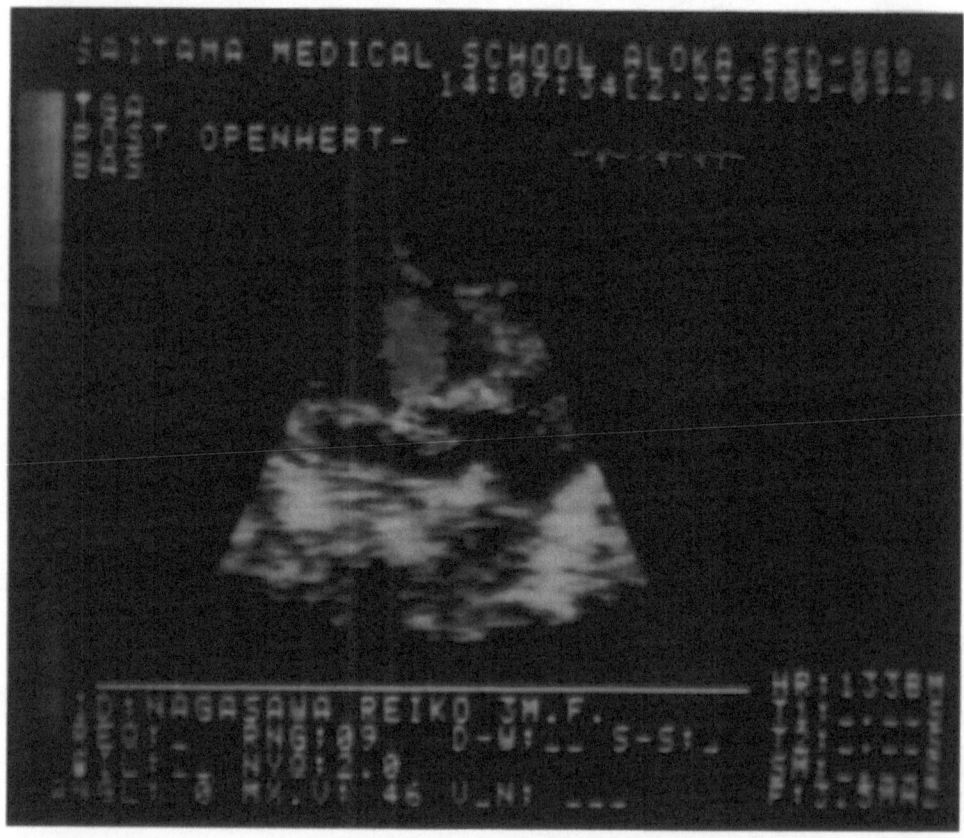

Figure 14. Two-dimensional color flow following septostomy. From subcostal approach, the right atrium is toward the top, left atrium toward the bottom, and the dense white interatrial septal echo is shown. A sizeable defect in the septal echo is replaced by orange colors which begin on the left side of the septum and extend into the right atrium, indicating left to right ASD flow. Examination performed by author at Saitama Medical School, Saitama Japan, courtesy Dr. Shunei Kyo.

Table 8. Severity of atrioventricular valve regurgitation.

	2D/Doppler	Brandestini	Aloka
None	10/10	10/10	8/10
Mild	4/5	5/5	4/5
Moderate	6/7	6/7	5/7
Severe	3/3	3/3	1/3
Agreement with ventriculogram	92%	96%	72%

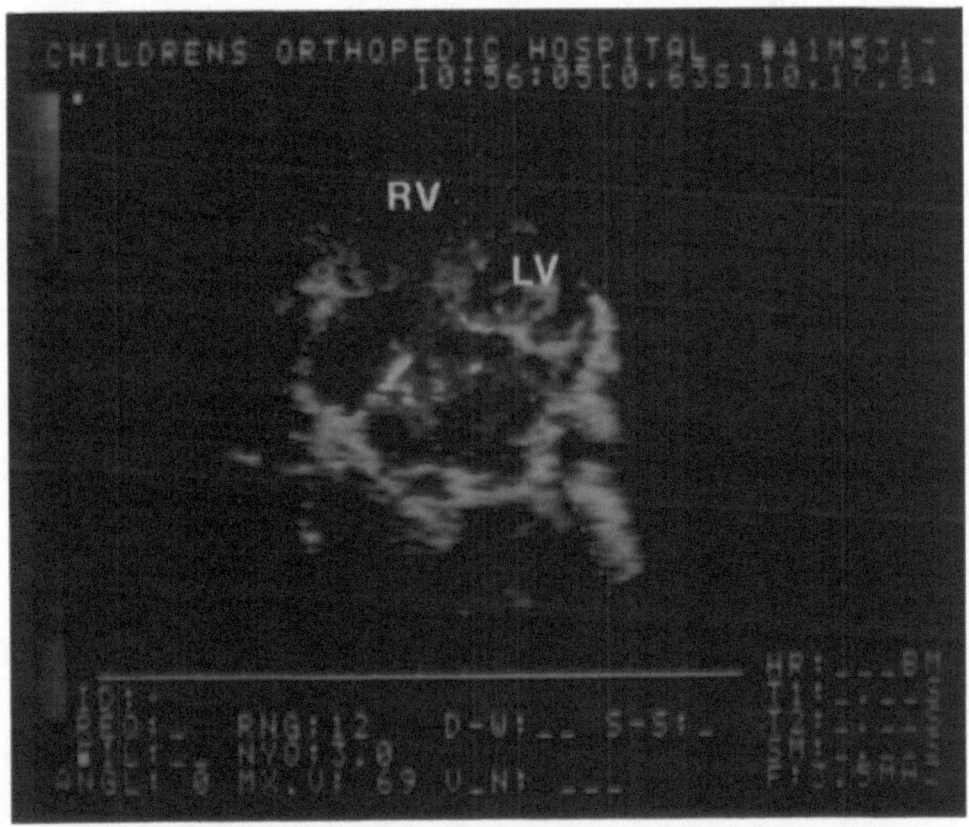

Figure 15. Two-dimensional color flow, ostium primum atrial septal defect with associated mitral regurgitation. Orientation is similar to Figure 13. The orange left to right primum ASD flow is evident. Posterior to the mitral valve is a blue jet of regurgitation.

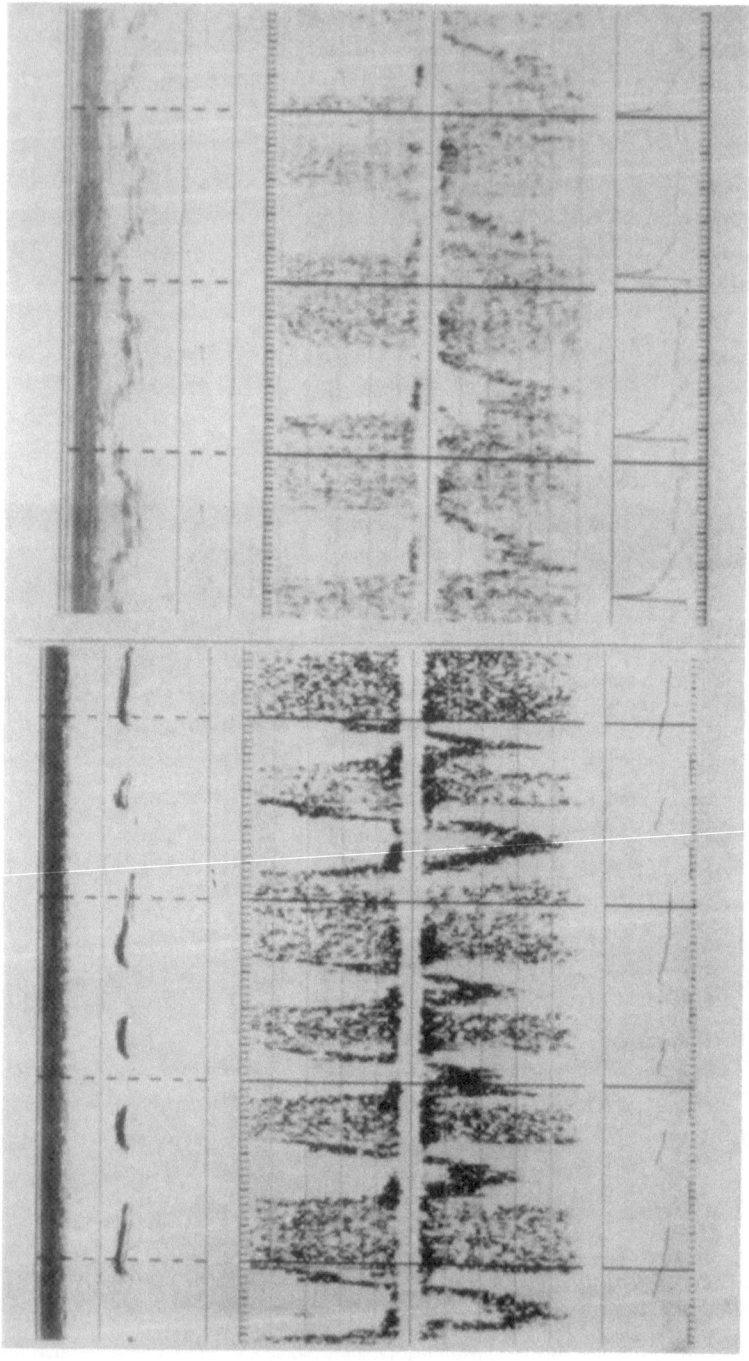

Figure 16. Conventional Doppler flow records of aortic regurgitation and of mitral stenosis. Both panels have been obtained from sample volume placement in the left ventricular outflow tract. On the left, with placement near the aortic valve, there is diastolic spectral broadening from aortic regurgitation. The other panel, from the mitral valve, shows diastolic turbulence and velocity of mitral stenosis. The waveforms are essentially indistinguishable.

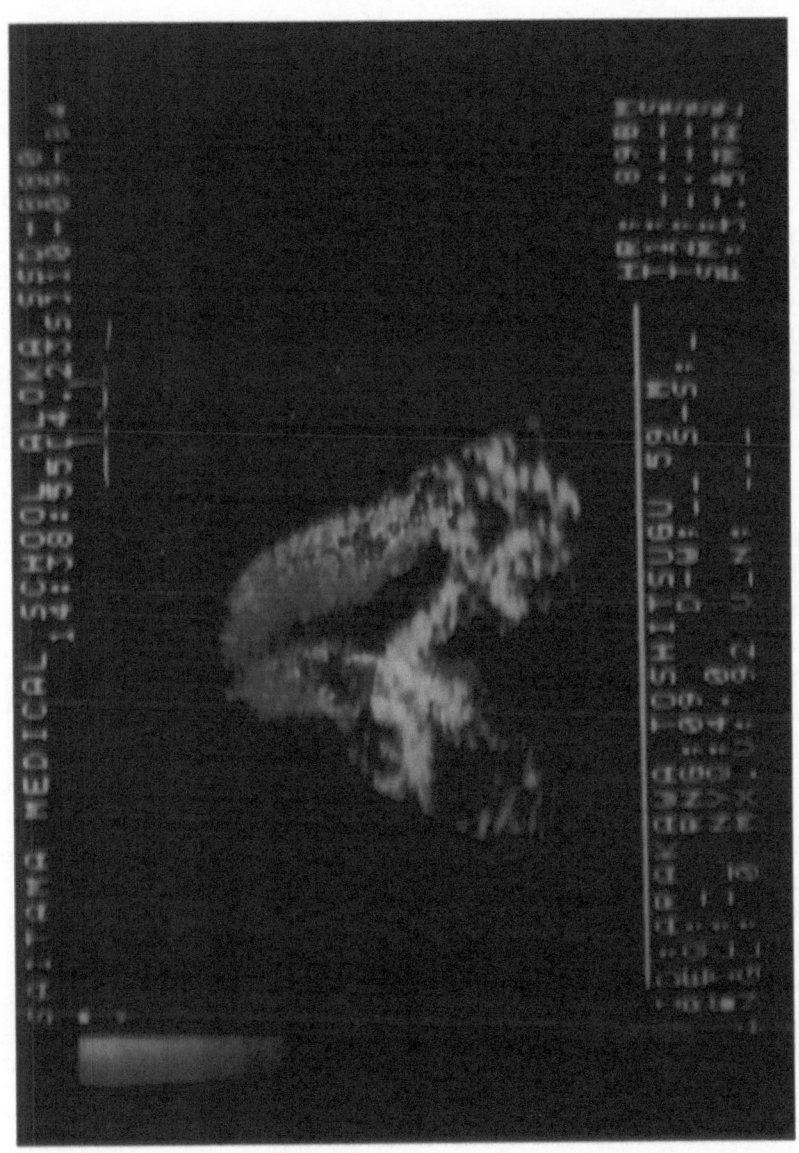

Figure 17. Two-dimensional color flow of mitral stenosis and aortic regurgitation. The aortic valve appears toward the right, and the domed stenotic mitral valve appears toward the left. From each valve, a peripherally orange jet (centrally blue from aliasing) extends into the left ventricular outflow tract. The course and boundaries of the two jets define two distinct flow disturbances. Examination performed by author at Saitama Medical School, Saitama, Japan. courtesy Dr. Shinichi Takamoto.

needs the capability to evaluate certain areas of interest while momentarily excluding confusing flow information coming from other areas. Some have used the M-mode color format as a means to sample flow, and then use the frozen display for thoughtful review and analysis. Imaging of flow across only a portion of the image is an alternative approach, as could be operator-controlled velocity display limits. The low two dimensional frame rate of currently available systems is a definite drawback; frame rate and image quality can only be expected to improve in future generations of equipment.

As Doppler and cardiac ultrasound have grown through the years, we have seen initially 'competing' ultrasound modalities come together into single systems wherein each modality can be used for a superior application; the combination of continuous wave with pulsed Doppler is an example. It is then likely that color flow will be added to the capabilities already present in conventional systems, leading to an ideal comprehensive Doppler instrument.

Acknowledgement

I have summarized the development and application of color flow imaging at our institutions; obviously it has been a team effort, with many members of the team. It is difficult to convey the depth of gratitude and respect for the knowledge, capability, patience and perseverance of my many engineering, medical, surgical and nursing colleagues and friends who have participated in this effort. It simply could not have been done, and cannot continue without this kind of cooperation and interchange. Equally deserving of recognition is the collaborative atmosphere which has surrounded the realization by each team that similar color flow approaches and problems, were being addressed on opposite sides of the Pacific. It is in the spirit of recognition and admiration of accomplishment that I have included figures in this chapter from examinations which I was fortunate to have been able to perform in the laboratories of several of our distinguished Japanese color flow colleagues.

References

1. Brandestini MA: Topoflow: a digital full range Doppler velocity meter. IEEE Son-Ultrason, SU25–5: 287–293, 1978.
2. Brandestini MA, Eyer MA, Stevenson JG: M/Q mode echocardiography: the synthesis of conventional echo with digital multigate Doppler, pp. 441–46. In: Lancee CT (ed.) Echocardiology. The Hague, Martinus Nijhoff: 1979.
3. Stevenson JG, Brandestini MA, Weiler T, Howard A, Eyer MA: Digital multigate Doppler with color echo and Doppler display: Diagnosis of atrial and ventricular septal defects. Circulation 60 (2): 205, 1979.
4. Brandestini MA, Howard A, Eyer MA, Stevenson JG, Weiler T: Visualization of intracardiac

defects by M/Q mode Echo/Doppler ultrasound. Circulation 60 (2): 12, 1979.

5. Stevenson JG, Kawabori I, Brandestini MA: A twenty month experience comparing conventional pulsed Doppler echocardiography and color coded digital multigate Doppler for detection of atrioventricular valve regurgitation and its severity. In: Rijsterborgh H (ed.) Echocardiology pp. 399–407. The Hague, Martinus Nijhoff: 1981.

6. Omoto R: Color atlas of real time two dimensional echocardiography. Tokyo, Shindan-to-Chiryo: 1984.

7. Stevenson JG, Kawabori I, Dooley TK, Guntheroth WG: Diagnosis of ventricular septal defect by pulsed Doppler echocardiography: Sensitivity, specificity and limitations. Circulation 58: 322–326, 1978.

8. Stevenson JG: Multigate Doppler evaluation of flow disturbances in congenital heart disease. In: Spencer M (ed.) Cardiac Doppler Diagnosis pp. 235–45. Boston: Martinus Nijhoff, 1983.

9. Stevenson JG, Kawabori I, Brandestini MA: Color coded visualization of flow within ventricular septal defects: Implications for peak pulmonary artery pressure. Am J Cardiology 49: 944, 1982.

10. Stevenson JG, Kawabori I, Guntheroth WG: Pulsed Doppler echocardiographic diagnosis of patent ductus arteriosus: Sensitivity, specificity. limitations and technical features. Catheterization and Cardiovascular Diagnosis 6: 255–263, 1980.

11. Gentile R, Stevenson JG, Dooley TK, Franklin D, Kawabori I, Pearlman AS: Pulsed Doppler echocardiographic determination of time of ductal closure in normal newborn infants. J. Pediatrics 98: 443–448, 1981.

12. Daniels O, Hopman JC, Stoelinga GB, Busch HJ, Peer PG: Doppler flow characteristics in the main pulmonary artery and the LA/AO ratio before and after ductal closure in healthy newborns. Pediatr Cardiol 3: 99–105, 1982.

13. Pearlman AS, Lighty GW, Jr: Clinical applications of two dimensional/pulsed Doppler echocardiography. Cardiovasc Clinics 13 (3), 201–238, 1983.

14. Sakakibara H, Miyatake K, Izumi S, Kinoshita N, Asonuma H, Nimura Y: Assessment of mitral and aortic regurgitation by real time two dimensional Doppler flow imaging system. Circulation 70–2: 406, 1984.

15. Asaka T, Yoshikawa J, Yoshida K, Koizumi F, Okumachi K, Yanagihara K, Kato H, Shiratori K: Sensitivity and specificity of real time two dimensional Doppler flow imaging system in the detection of valvar regurgitation. Circulation 70–2: 38, 1984.

16. Stevenson JG, Kawabori I: Sequential 2D/Echo-Doppler: Improved diagnosis of atrial septal defect. Circulation 68–4: 110, 1983.

17. Kyo S, Omoto R, Takamoto S, Takanawa E: Quantitative estimation of intracardiac shunt flow in atrial septal defect by real time two dimensional color flow Doppler. Circulation 70–2: 39, 1984.

18. Bommer WJ, Rebeck K, Laviola S, LaFranchise L, Jackson T, Keown M: Real time two dimensional flow imaging: Detection and semiquantitation of valvular and congenital heart disease. Circulation 70–2: 38, 1984.

Does color flow mapping Doppler echocardiography allow the catheterization laboratory to be bypassed in surgery of congenital heart disease?

Shunei Kyo, Shinichi Takamoto, Eiko Takanawa, Makoto Matsumura,
Yuji Yokote and Ryozo Omoto

Abstract

The purpose of this study is to demonstrate the clinical usefulness of color flow mapping real-time two-dimensional Doppler echocardiography (2-D Doppler) in establishing the diagnosis of congenital heart disease (CHD) and its application for intraoperative use. In the past two years we examined a series of 278 patients (pts) with CHD including 97 infants and 105 children. With this device, real-time two-dimensional intracardiac and major vascular blood flow images on B-mode echocardiography have been clearly displayed by red color (flow towards the transducer) and blue color (flow away from the transducer) mixed with green color (variance of blood flow velocity) and graded brightness (average blood flow velocity). Patients suffered from ASD (75 pts), VSD (76 pts), TOF (23 pts), TGA (12 pts), PDA (23 pts), ECD (13 pts), PS (13 pts) or miscellaneous CHD, (47 pts). These diagnoses were confirmed by cardiac catheterization and/or surgery with the exception of PDA in premature infants. In 271 patients (97%) abnormal intracardiac blood flow (shunt flow, stenotic flow, and regurgitant flow) was clearly visualized by 2-D Doppler. In 31 patients several palliative procedures (Blalock-Taussig shunt operation: 8, Brock operation: 2, pulmonary arterial banding: 10, BAS: 11) were performed mostly based on 2-D Doppler diagnosis. Fifteen premature infants with PDA and respiratory failure were followed up using 2-D Doppler during Sulindac (prostaglandin antagonist) therapy and 3 infants resistent to Sulindac therapy underwent surgery. In 10 patients intraoperative 2-D Doppler evaluations were performed for confirmation of the diagnosis, confirmation of the completeness of surgery, and for 2-D Doppler echo guided blade atrioseptostomy by direct right atrial approach in the case of d-TGA with bilateral iliac venous obstraction. In conclusion, 2-D Doppler diagnosis was satisfactory in about 90% of corrective surgical cases. Therefore, 2-D Doppler can be a useful non-invasive diagnostic tool for CHD. Also, 2-D Doppler is effective for intraoperative evaluation of multiple cardiac abnormalities in complex CHD and for confirmation of the completeness of surgery. It is suggested that surgery can be carried out without cardiac catheterization in a significant number of congenital heart diseases.

Introduction

The major advantage of color flow mapping real-time Doppler echocardiography (2-D Doppler) in the cardiovascular disease is the possibility it offers to evaluate the abnormal intracardiac circulation and the anatomical abnormalities of the diseases simultaneously in real-time [1, 2]. With real-time color flow mapping of intracardiac blood flow, 2-D Doppler has a potential feasibility to assess the abnormal intracardiac blood flow quantitatively [3]. Also, the current commercial model (Aloka SSD-880) contains M-mode color flow mapping function, fast Fourier transformation (FFT) pulsed Doppler spectral analysis function, and continuous wave Doppler (CW Doppler) function. Therefore, it allows the evaluation of the intracardiac abnormal blood flow more precisely, qualitatively and quantitatively. With these advantages 2-D Doppler allows a definitive anatomical and physiological diagnosis to be made in many cases of complex congenital heart disease [4, 5, 6].

For critically ill patients the determination of indications for surgical treatment in appropriate timing is most important for saving the patients life. For that sake they have to undergo cardiac catheterization repeatedly. However, catheterization itself is significantly related to mortality and morbidity of critically ill patients [7]. Therefore, we have been seeking an adequate non-invasive diagnostic tool for these patients. 2-D Doppler has potential use in directing medical or surgical management of patients and changing the indication for cardiac catheterization, especially in the emergent case of newborn or infant severe cardio-respiratory failure. In this chapter we review our two years experience of color flow mapping real-time Doppler echocardiography in congenital heart disease and we demonstrate the clinical significance of this new technology in patient management. We also discuss to what extent we can bypass the cardiac catheterization laboratory in the determination of surgical indications for congenital heart disease by using 2-D Doppler diagnostically and intraoperatively [8, 9].

Materials

2-D Doppler examination was performed at Saitama Medical School on 278 patients with congenital heart disease and 87 children with anatomically normal hearts in the foregoing 28 months (Jan. 1983 – April 1985). In the group of congenital heart disease 97 infants, 105 children, and 76 adult cases were included (Table 1). The diagnosis of 278 cases of congenital heart disease was established and confirmed by cardiac catheterization and/or by direct evaluation during

Table 1.

Diseases	Infant	Child	Adult	Total
ASD	12	25	38	75
VSD	31	31	15	76
TOF	7	11	15	23
TGA	10	2	0	12
PDA	15*	5	3	23
PS, PA	4	8	1	13
ECD	7	2	4	13
Others	12	21	10	43
Total	97	105	76	278

ASD = atrial septal defect, VSD = ventricular septal defect, TOF = tetralogy of Fallot, TGA = transposition of great arteries, PDA = patent ductus arteriosus, PS = pulmonary stenosis, PA = pure pulmonary atresia, ECD = endocardial cushion defect.
* Premature infants: Cath. examination (−) (Jan. 1983–Apr. 1985, at SMS).

open chest surgery with the exception of 15 cases of patent ductus arteriosus in premature infants. The population of normal hearts included 25 patients with a history of Kawasaki disease, 16 premature infants with heart murmur, 11 children with heart murmur, and 35 clinically normal children. Among 278 patients with congenital heart disease 83 patients underwent corrective surgery and 31 patients underwent palliative surgery. Among 87 children with normal hearts 25 patients with a history of Kawasaki disease and 11 children with heart murmur had not been detected as being cardiac abnormal by cardiac catheterization. Also, 16 premature infants in the normal group took a normal clinical course and their heart murmur had disappeared before discharge from the hospital.

Intraoperative 2-D Doppler evaluation was performed in 10 patients, including 2 atrial septal defects (ASD), 3 ventricular septal defects (VSD), 1 total anormalus pulmonary venous connection (TAPVC), 1 transposition of great arteries (d-TGA), 1 coronary arterio-venous fistula, 1 cor triatrium with large VSD, and 1 reoperation case of tetralogy of Fallot (TOF). In 8 cases corrective surgery was performed, in one case of d-TGA a palliative operative atrioseptostomy was performed, and in one case of VSD with congestive heart failure a pulmonary arterial banding surgery (PA-banding) was performed.

Methods

We obtained color flow mapping Doppler echocardiograms using the XA-54, the SSD-880, and the XA-340 produced by Aloka Co. Ltd. Tokyo, Japan (Table 2). Th XA-54 and the SSD-880 have a phased-array sector scanner utilizing a

Table 2. 2D-Doppler instruments.

Aloka XA-54	2.5 MHz, 3.0 MHz, 3.5 MHz
Aloka SSD-880	2.5 MHz, 3.5 MHz
Aloka XA-340	5.0 MHz, 7.5 MHz
Flow towards the transducer	red
Flow away from the transducer	blue
Variance of velocity	mixture of green
Velocity measurement	FFT spectral analysis
	CW Doppler

FFT = fast Fourier transformation, CW = continuous wave.

transducer with 2.5, 3.0, 3.5 MHz frequency and 4, 6, 8 KHz repetition frequency. The XA-340, a special model for intraoperative use, has a linear-array scanner with a convex type transducer of 5 MHz frequency and a linear type transducer of 7.5 MHz frequency. Repetition frequency of XA-340 are 2 and 4 KHz. We have already described the basic color flow display pattern of these instruments. Minimal velocity displayed in color is about 10 cm/sec in XA-54 and SSD-880, and 2 cm/sec in XA-340. Before intraoperative use the transducer was gas sterilized by the ethylene oxide technique for at least 24 hours. Before operation informed consent was obtained in the case of intraoperative use of 2-D Doppler. No arrhythmia or other complications related to intraoperative 2-D Doppler were noted.

Results

In 271 patients (97%) of 278 studied cases of congenital heart disease, we could visualize intracardiac abnormal blood flow in association with anatomical abnormalities. We failed to visualize the abnormal intracardiac blood flow in 7 patients. They were two adult cases and one premature infant case (1100 g of body weight when 14 days old) of patent ductus arteriosus, one adult case and one child case of secundum type ASD, one adult case of sinus venosus type ASD, and one adult case of TOF with dextrocardia. Among 202 cases of pediatric congenital heart disease we failed to visualize the abnormal intracardiac blood flow in 2 cases (1%).

Among the 87 cases of the normal heart group, only 8 premature infants demonstrated transient small abnormal shunt flow through patent foramen ovale.

Corrective surgery was performed on 83 cases and palliative procedure was performed on 31 cases as shown in Table 3. Seven corrective surgeries were performed without cardiac catheterization: 5 of them were ligation closures of the patent ductus arteriosus (PDA) of premature infants or newborn. One case was

Table 3. Surgical case.

Corrective surgery		Palliative surgery	
VSD	16 (1)	Pa-banding	10 (3)
ASD	43 (1)	Brock Op.	2 (1)
PDA	11 (5)	Shunt Op.	8 (4)
TOF	3	BAS	11 (11)
TGA	2		
AS, AR	2		
PS, PA	2		
Others	4		
	83 (7)		31 (19)

VSD = ventricular septal defect, ASD = atrial septal defect, PDA = patent ductus arteriosus, TOF = tetralogy of Fallot, TGA = transposition of great arteries, AS = aortic stenosis, AR = aortic regurgitation, PS = pulmonary stenosis, PA = pulmonary atresia, PA-banding = pulmonary arterial banding, BAS = balloon atrioseptostomy.
( ): Noncatheterization case before surgery

that of a 20-year-old male who, suffering from infectious endocarditis with a small membranous VSD, developed septicemia and tricuspid valve vegetation. VSD direct suture closure and tricuspid valve replacement was performed on this case. The other case was an ASD of a 13 year-old-boy who had an allergic reaction to radiographic contrast material.

Thirty-one premature infants with heart murmur were examined by 2-D Doppler in their early stage of life and 2-D Doppler demonstrated an obvious shunt flow through patent ductus arteriosus in 15 cases. In 12 cases PDA was closed spontaneously or after medical therapy. However, in 3 cases a persistent PDA shunt flow was observed even after a series of Sulindac (prostaglandin antagonist) therapy and their respiratory failure had advanced, so surgical closure of the ductus arteriosus was performed. Figure 1 demonstrates the clinical course of one surgical case (gestational age: 38th week, birth weight: 2500 g).

Nineteen palliative procedures were performed without cardiac catheterization. In three cases of VSD with pulmonary hypertension PA-banding was performed without preoperative cardiac catheterization. In these 3 cases 2-D Doppler demonstrated a relatively increased main pulmonary arterial blood flow and a decreased velocity of shunt flow through the ventricular septal defect. Therefore, the color flow pattern of the shunt flow was not a mosaic pattern and the shunt flow velocity was smaller than 2.5 m/sec in these 3 cases. In one case a Brock operation, in two cases a Blalock-Taussig shunt operation, and in two cases a central shunt operation using Gore-Tex graft was performed simply depending on clinical manifestation and 2-D Doppler diagnosis. In four cases of shunt operation preoperative 2-D Doppler demonstrated a decreased blood flow

112

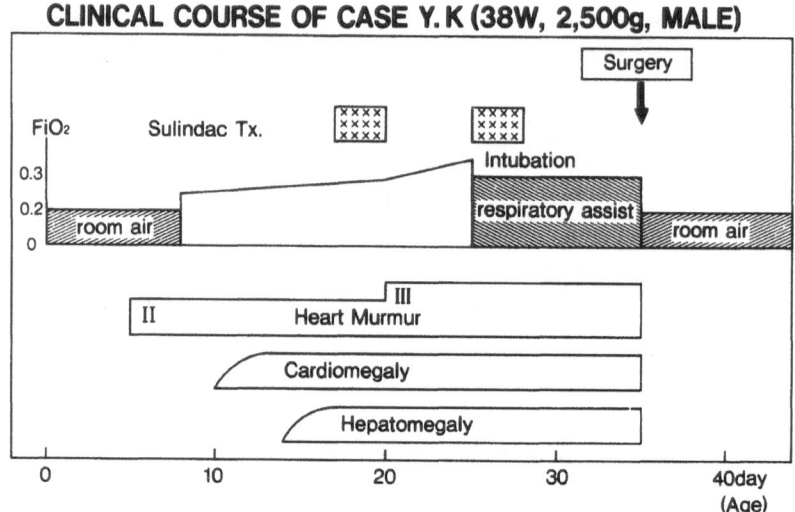

CLINICAL COURSE OF CASE Y. K (38W, 2,500g, MALE)

Figure 1. The clinical course in the premature infant case of patent ductus arteriosus (PDA). In this case two series of Sulindac (prostagrandin antagonist) therapy was not effective and cardio-respiratory failure was advanced. 2-D Doppler demonstrated a high flow isolate PDA, then surgical intervention was performed at 35th day after birth.

in the main pulmonary artery and the pulmonary arterial branches. Eleven balloon and/or blade atrioseptostomies (BAS) were performed under 2-D Doppler echo-guide. In 9 cases the preoperative diagnosis was established by 2-D Doppler immediately after hospitalization as being d-TGA in 6 cases, tricuspid atresia in 2 cases, and pure pulmonary atresia in one case. Second blade and balloon atrioseptostomy was performed in two cases of d-TGA due to re-narrowing of the interatrial opening (IAO) at 2 and 7 months after the first BAS. In one of these cases operative BAS with a small right anterior thoracotomy was performed as a substitute for the Blalock-Hanlon operation. Figure 2 demonstrates the re-narrowing of the interatrial opening and the decreased shunt flow through IAO in the subxiphoid four-chamber view of this case. After BAS we were able to confirm, using 2-D Doppler, that a moderate size of IAO and a sufficient shunt flow through IAO were obtained in this case.

In 76 cases corrective surgery and in 12 cases a palliative procedure was performed after full 2-D Doppler echocardiographic and full cardiac catheterization examination. In 6 of these 88 cases (6.8%) we could not obtain diagnostic information from the 2-D Doppler examination. Although we could obtain diagnostic information by 2-D Doppler in 3 other cases (3.4%), it was not satisfactory to perform a corrective surgery, because we could not detect the azygos connection and the persistent left superior vena cava in one case of cor triatriatum with VSD and also we could not detect the associated partial anomalous pulmonary venous connection in two cases of ASD. Therefore, when review-

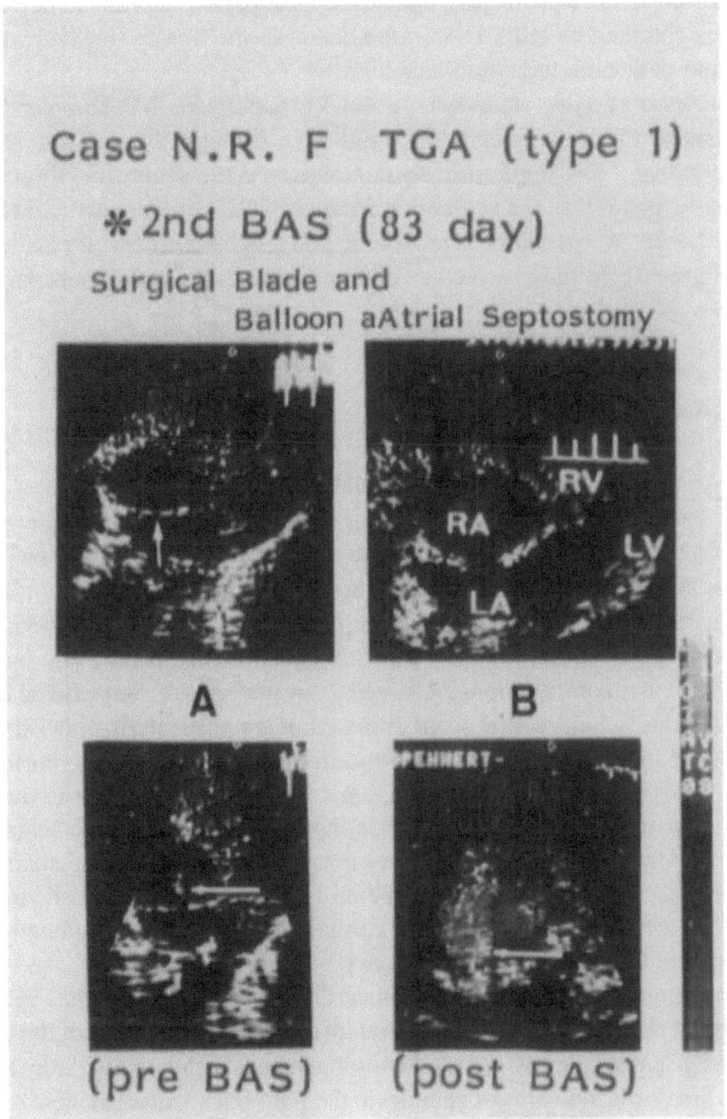

Figure 2. A: 2-D Doppler demonstrated a re-narrowing of interatrial opening (IAO) and decreased shunt flow through it. B: After blade and balloon atrioseptostomy (BAS) 2-D Doppler demonstrated a moderate size of IAO and a sufficient shunt flow through it. RV = right ventricle. LA = left atrium, LV = left ventricle.

ing retrospectively, satisfactory diagnostic information in order to perform surgery was obtained by full 2-D Doppler diagnosis in 79 cases (89.8%) which was consistent with catheterization diagnosis.

In the case of sinus venosus-type ASD preoperative 2-D Doppler failed to demonstrate the defects and the shunt flow through the defects. However, intraoperative 2-D Doppler clearly demonstrated the shunt flow through sinus venosus-type ASD. In the re-operation case of TOF intraoperative 2-D Doppler demonstrated two portions of prosthetic patch dehiscences with residual shunt flow (Figure 3). In these two cases intraoperative 2-D Doppler was particularly effective.

Discussion

Cardiac catheterization has been the standard means of diagnosing most congenital heart diseases which can establish not only anatomical abnormalities but also blood flow and pressure hemodynamics qualitatively and quantitatively. However, as an invasive diagnostic technique cardiac catheterization entails several complications [10]: local vascular complications, arrhythmia and conduction disturbance, perforation of the heart and great vessels, myocardial infarction, cerebrovascular complications. Also, contrast material-related cardiac dysfunction, respiratory failure, and renal dysfunction are particularly noticeable in the critically ill infants. Although it is associated with morbidity and mortality, we have to perform cardiac catheterization repeatedly in some cases during the course of patient management because the alterations in cardiac anatomy and hemodynamics are very rapid in the newborn and infant. Therefore, many efforts have been focussed on the establishment of a non-invasive diagnostic technique which can totally replace the role of cardiac catheterization including real-time visualization of intracardiac blood flow [11–14].

Conventional two-dimensional echocardiography (2-D Echo) has become an established non-invasive diagnostic tool for anatomical diagnosis of the congenital heart disease. Contrast-assisted two-dimensional echocardiography has been used to assess the blood flow dynamics in the right side cardiac cavities. Also, CW Doppler and pulsed wave Doppler echocardiographic techniques were introduced to evaluate the intracardiac and major vascular blood circulation. However, the technique for CW Doppler and pulsed wave Doppler echocardiography may be diffcult in respect to the determination of the spatial orientation of flow, and, therefore, in defining the location of the areas where abnormal flows exist [15]. Also, in terms of quantification of abnormal intracardiac flow, we cannot accomplish the real-time flow mapping by these techniques. The impact of color flow mapping real-time two-dimensional Doppler echocardiography is that we can obtain the real-time distribution of normal and abnormal intracardiac blood flow with simultaneous two-dimensional echocardiograms. This new technology

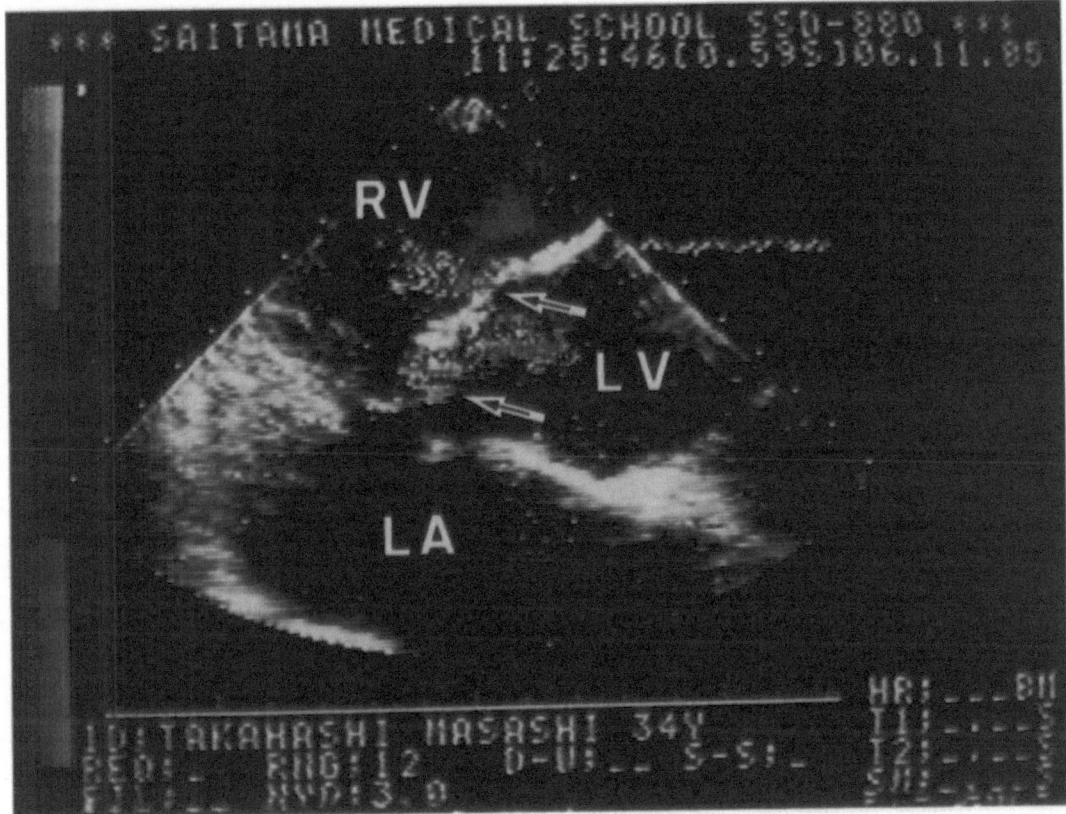

Figure 3. Intraoperative 2-D Doppler demonstrated two ventricular septal defect (VSD) in the re-operation case of TOF. The size of VSDs were 1 mm (the upper VSD) and 8 mm (the lower VSD) at surgery.

is especially useful in the evaluation of hemodynamics in the small heart of infants, premature infants, and fetuses within reasonably short time, usually less than 15 minutes [16, 17].

With this device, to what extent can we perform surgeries without cardiac catheterization? In the case of an atrial septal defect (ASD), we have already demonstrated the usefulness of the maximum shunt flow area index (MSFAI) for the quantitative estimation of the shunt ratio by 2-D Doppler [3]. Maximum shunt flow area (MSFA) can be obtained using a slow-motion play-back technique of a videotape of a recorded 2-D Doppler shunt flow image through ASD in the standard parasternal or apical four-chamber view. For normalization MSFA was corrected for body surface area (BSA); the MSFAI was calculated by MSFA/BSA. A good correlation between shunt ratio (SR) estimated by cardiac catheterization and MSFAI was observed (Figure 4). When the shunt ratio exceeds 33% ($Qp/Qs = 1.5$) in the case of ASD it is considered as a surgical indication [18]. In

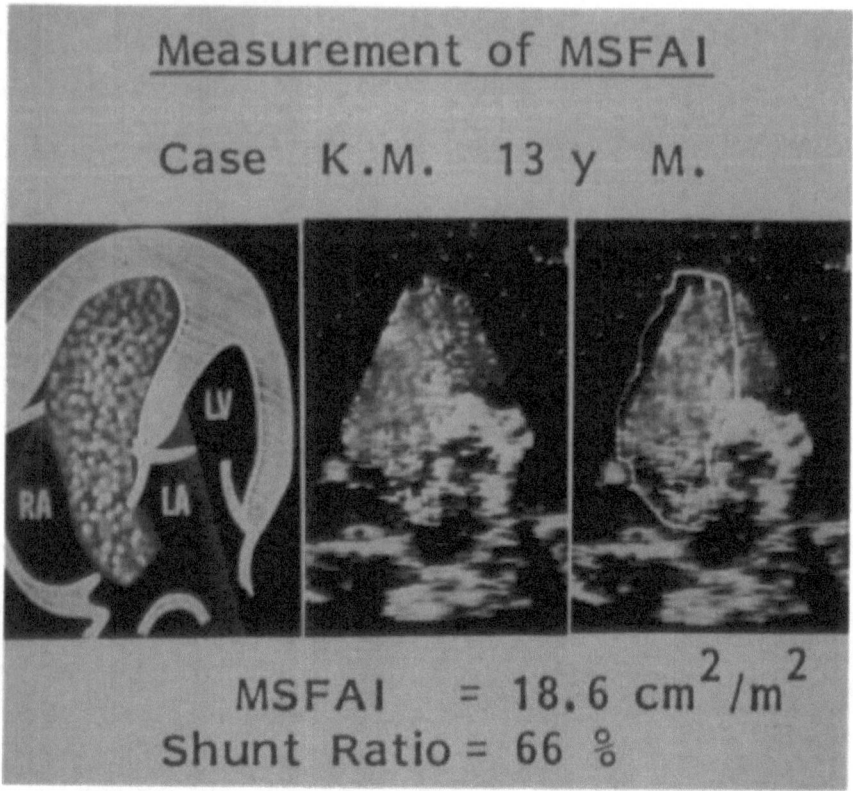

Figure 4. This atrial septal defect (ASD) case was performed surgery without cardiac catheterization due to allergic reaction to radiographic contrast material. From maximum shunt flow area index (MSFAI) the shunt ratio was estimated as 66% by 2-D Doppler. The blood sampling at surgery deonstrated the shunt ratio as 73%. RA = right atrium, LA = left atrium, LV = left ventricle.

our series when 2-D Doppler demonstrated MSFAI more than $10\,cm^2/m^2$ the shunt ratio obtained by cardiac catheterization demonstrated more than 40% and all these ASD cases were considered to be a candidate for surgery. Also, 2-D Doppler is effective in the detection of secondary associated valvular lesions. Eleven of the studied ASD cases were accompanied by mitral regurgitation, tricuspid regurgitation, or both regurgitations. When we observe these associated secondary valvular lesions 2-D Doppler is also useful in the determination of the surgical indication and the required surgical procedure.

When the PDA is first encountered in large centers operative intervention is suggested in all children, symptomatic or asymptomatic [19]. Therefore, in the case of isolated PDA when the diagnosis of PDA is established and confirmed by 2-D Doppler we consider that surgery can be performed without cardiac catheterization. We did not experience any difficulty in diagnosing PDA in pediatric cases; however, we have failed to demonstrate the PDA shunt flow in two of three adult PDA cases. In the adult case of PDA the left lung often prevents the Doppler echo penetration to the main pulmonary artery by the standard precordial approach. In such a case the transesophagial approach can be a potent diagnostic approach. VSD patients with small defects (Qp/Qs less than 1.5 and normal pulmonary pressure) require no surgical treatment and VSD patients with moderate to large defects are considered to be surgical candidates [20]. Earlier surgical closure is recommended for VSD patients with pulmonary hypertension in which the pulmonary resistance (PR) is elevated more than 5 units/m^2 in order to prevent irreversible pulmonary vascular change. In this study we experienced 12 cases of isolated VSD with severely increased pulmonary vascular resistance (PR greater than 8 units/m^2). All 12 cases demonstrated large VSD with a decreased velocity of VSD shunt flow measured by FFT spectral analysis or CW Doppler. Therefore, the color flow mapping pattern of VSD shunt flow was not a mosaic pattern but rather a simple color flow pattern [21]. Their VSD shunt flow velocity was lower than 2.5 m/sec by CW Doppler measurement. In 4 cases 2-D Doppler demonstrated bi-directional and multi-phasic VSD shunt flow pattern. Two cases of them were diagnosed Eisenmenger VSD by 2-D Doppler and cardiac catheterization. Figure 5 demonstrates B-mode 2-D Echo and M-mode 2-D Doppler of Eisenmenger VSD in a 20-year-old male. In this case M-mode 2-D Doppler demonstrated a bi-directional and quadriphasic shunt flow pattern and the time interval of right to left shunt (displayed in blue) is almost equal to that of left to right shunt (displayed in red) in the cardiac cycle (Figure 5 (B)). We decided that surgery was contraindicated in this case. Figure 6 demonstrates another case of VSD with pulmonary hypertension of a four-year-old female. This case also demonstrated a bi-directional an bi-phasic shunt flow pattern in M-mode 2-D Doppler. However, looking at the time interval of left to right shunt (displayed in red) in the cardiac cycle we observe that it is longer than the time interval of right to left shunt (displayed in blue) (Figure 6 (B)). Although cardiac catheterization demonstrated a typical hemodynamics which is compatible to Eisenmenger VSD (Figure 6 (A)), we determined this case to be an indication for surgery depending on the 2-D Doppler diagnosis. Surgical correction was performed successfully and pulmonary arterial pressure was decreased dramatically after patch closure of VSD. It may be difficult to determine the surgical indication by 2-D Doppler alone in the case of mild to moderate VSD, because this technique does not provide a reliable, effective method to assess the grade of VSD shunt flow quantitatively. However, in the case of large VSD, especially in the case with advanced pulmonary hypertension, 2-D Doppler is useful in the determination of the surgical indication.

The palliative procedure was performed without cardiac catheterization in this study. All of these palliative surgical cases were infants in 19 of the 31 cases (61.3%) and resolution of 2-D Doppler is fairly good especially in the case of infants, which most apt to require an emergent palliative procedure. Therefore, it may be possible to determine the indication for all palliative procedures by 2-D

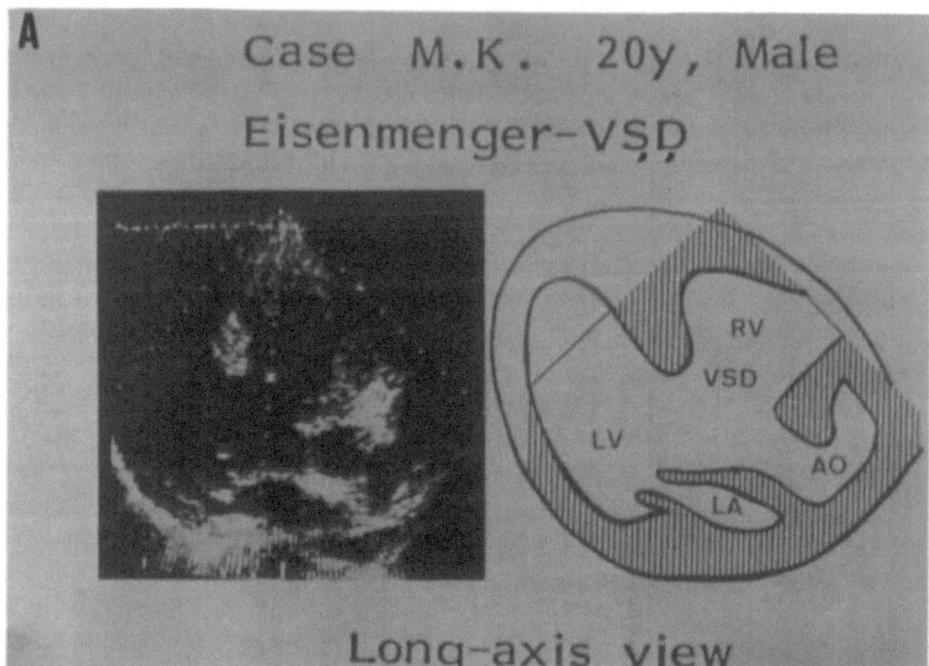

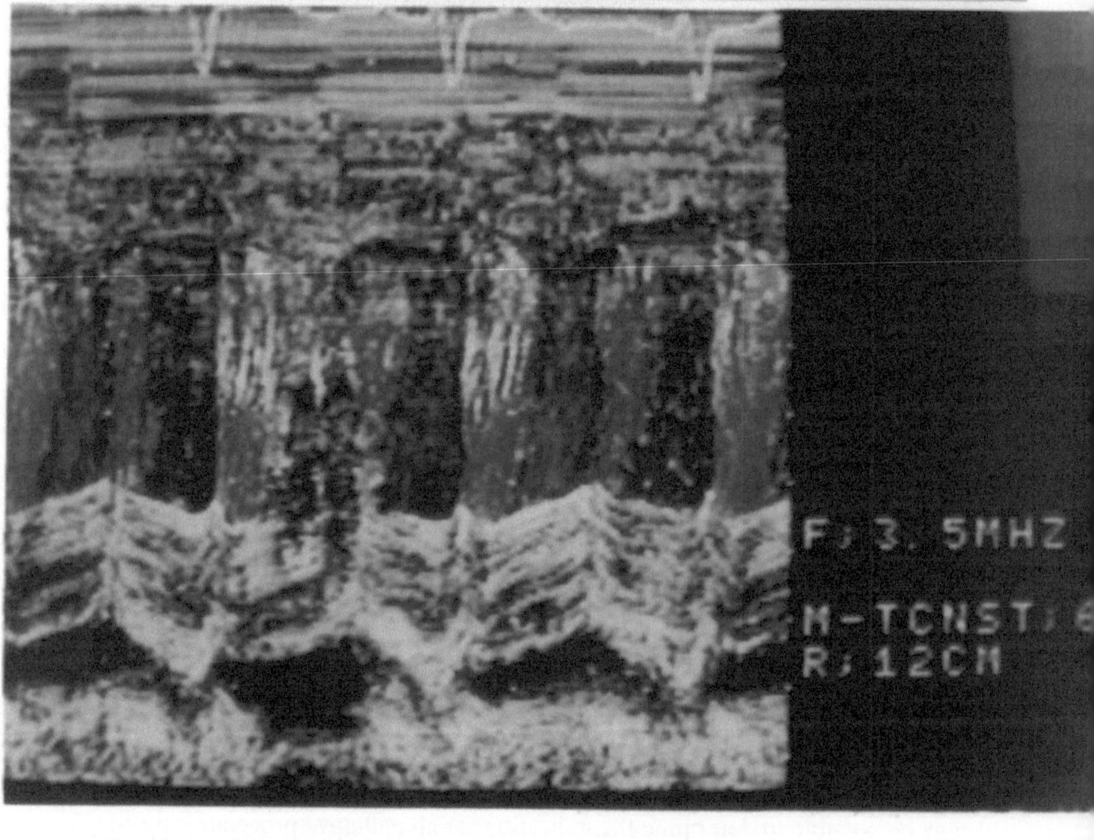

Figure 5. A: A large ventricular septal defect (VSD) was demonstrated in the standard long-axis view. B: M-mode sampled at the center of VSD demonstrates bi-directional and quadri-phasic shunt flow pattern which is considered to be compatible with cardiac catheterization.

Case M.M. 4 y.o Female

VSD + PH

★ Cath. Data

	Pressure (mmHg)	Sat. O2 (%)
RA	m=4.0	67
RV	110/0 (edp 3)	75
mPA	115/70 (m=85)	77
LV	110/0 (edp 1.5)	88
Fem. A	105/72 (m=95)	90
Shunt	lt. ➤ rt. 34.5 %	
	rt. ➤ lt. 27.6 %	

★ Effect of VSD Closure

	Pre-Op.	Post-Op.
Ao	75/45 mmHg	90/60 mmHg
PA	75/45 mmHg	33/17 mmHg
Ao flow	1.3 l/min.	2.1 l/min.
PA flow	5.5 l/min.	2.0 l/min.

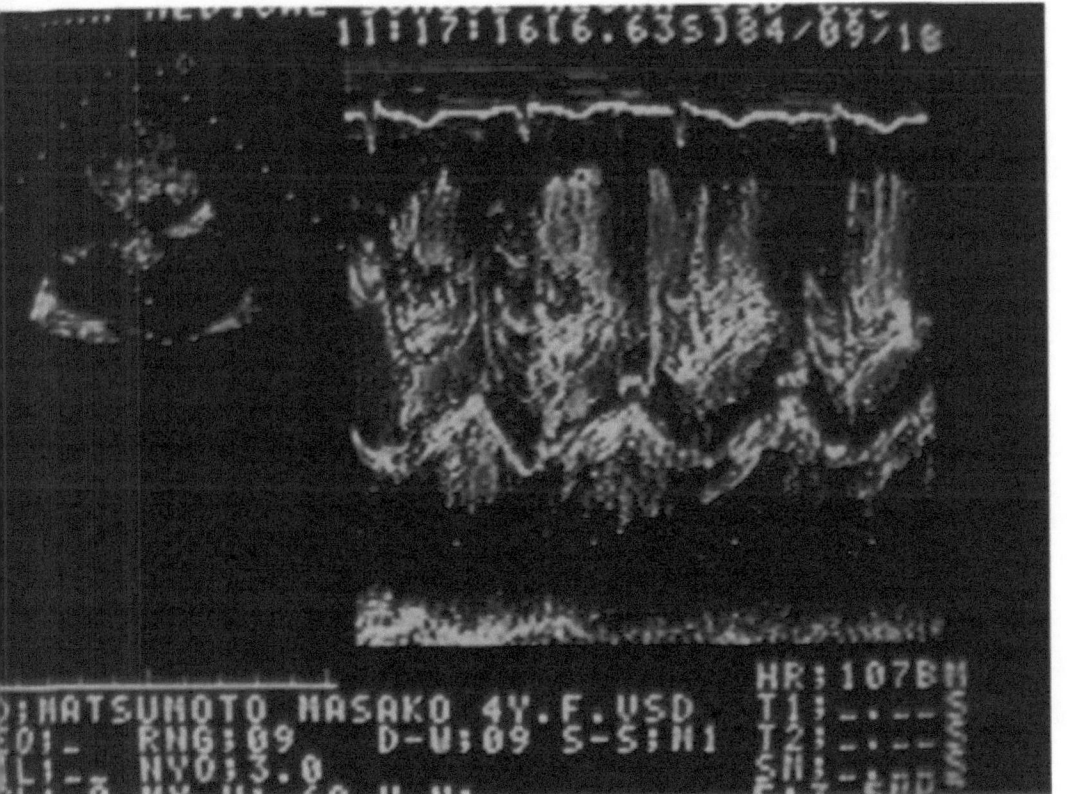

Figure 6. A: The preoperative cardiac catheterization data in the case of ventricular septal defect (VSD) demonstrates a bidirectional shunt and this case was suspected as a Eisenmenger VSD. RA = right atrium, RV = right ventricle, mPA = main pulmonary artery, LV = left ventricle, Fem. A = femoral artery, Ao = aorta, Sat. O₂ = oxygen saturation. B: However, M-mode 2-D Doppler demonstrates that the direction of the major part of the shunt flow is left to right displayed in red as a flow towards the transducer. By 2-D Doppler this case was considered to be an indication for surgery. A: After VSD closure Pulmonary arterial pressure was effectively decreased.

120

Doppler alone if necessary. Echo-guide balloon atrioseptostomy was introduced by Perry in 1981; we reported 2-D Doppler echo-guide balloon atrioseptostomy in 1985. Using 2-D Doppler we determine the diagnosis and indication, and we perform balloon atrioseptostomy under 2-D Doppler. In the patient follow-up 2-D Doppler is also useful to confirm the effects of BAS.

Our studied population contains a rather small number of complex heart disease, however, when we review the studied cases retrospectively, almost 90% of corrective surgery could be performed without cardiac catheterization. With intraoperative 2-D Doppler examination we can minimize the risk of overlooking the multiple lesion and associated lesion even if we bypass the preoperative cardiac catheterization.

Conclusions

2-D Doppler can be an useful non-invasive diagnostic tool for congenital heart disease and preoperative 2-D Doppler information has been satisfactory in 90% of corrective surgical cases.

Intraoperative 2-D Doppler is effective for detection and evaluation of the associated cardiac abnormalities in complex CHD and confirmation of the completeness of surgery.

It is suggested that surgery can be carried out without cardiac catheterization in a significant number of patients with congenital heart disease.

References

1. Omoto R, Yokote Y, Takamoto S, Kyo S, Ueda K, Asano H, Namekawa K, Kasai C, Kondo Y, Koyano A: The development of real-time two-dimensional Doppler echocardiography and its clinical significance in acquired valvular disease. With special reference to the evaluation of valvular regurgitation. Jpn Heart J 25: 325–340, 1984.
2. Omoto R (ed.): Color atlas of real-time two-dimensional Doppler echocardiography. Tokyo: Shindan-to-Chiryo, 1984 (distributed Lea & Febiger, Philadelphia).
3. Kyo S, Omoto R, Takamoto S, Takanawa E: Quantitative estimation of intracardiac shunt flow in atrial septal defect by real-time two-dimensional color flow Doppler. Circulation 70 (Suppl II): II–39, 1984.
4. Kyo S, Takamoto S, Ueda K, Emoto H, Tamura F, Asano H, Yokote Y, Omoto R, Takanawa E: Clinical significance of newly developed real-time two-dimensional Doppler echocardiography (2-D Doppler) in congenital heart diseases. With special reference to the assessment of intracardiac shunts. Proceedings of JSUA 43: 465–466, 1983.
5. Kyo S, Omoto R, Takamoto S, Ueda K, Emoto H, Asano H, Yokote Y: Real-time two-dimensional Doppler echocardiography (2-D Doppler) in congenital heart disease. Its clinical significance. J Cardiography 14: 785–801, 1984.
6. Kyo S, Omoto R, Takamoto S, Takanawa E: Clinical significance of color flow mapping real-time two-dimensional Doppler echocardiography (2-D Doppler) in congenital heart disease. Circulation 70 (Suppl II): II–37, 1984.

7. Rice MJ, Seward JB, Hagler DJ, Mair DD, Feldt RH, Puga FJ, Danielson GK, William DE, Tajik AJ: Impact of 2-dimensional echocardiography on the management of distressed newborns in whom cardiac disease is suspected. Am J Cardiol 51: 288–292, 1983.

8. Takamoto S, Kondo Y, Yoshikawa Y, Kasai C, Koyano A, Kyo S, Yokote Y, Omoto R: The first clinical experience of intraoperative real-time two-dimensional Doppler echocardiography in the dissecting aneurysm of the aorta. Proceedings of AIUM 29: 167, 1984.

9. Takamoto S, Kyo S, Yokote Y, Omoto R, sponsored by Buckley MJ: Intraoperative color flow mapping by real-time two-dimensional Doppler echocardiography for evaluation of the valvular and the congenital heart disease, and the vascular disease (Abstract). Program of Annual Meeting of 65th Am Assoc Thorac Surg: 32, 1985.

10. Grossman W: Complication of cardiac catheterization. Indication, causes and prevention. In: Grossman R (ed.) Cardiac catheterization and angiography, pp. 25–35. Philadelphia: Lea & Febiger, 1974.

11. Brandestini MA, Howard EA, Weile EB, Stevenson JG, Eyer MK: The synthesis of echo and Doppler in M-mode and sector scan. Proceedings of AIUM paper, No. 704: 125, 1979.

12. Kitabatake K, Inoue M, Asano M, Mishima M, Tanouchi J, Masuyama T, Hori M, Abe H, Chihara K, Sakurai H, Senda S, Morita H, Matsuo H: Non-invasive visualization of intracardiac blood flow in human heart using computer-aided pulsed Doppler technique. Clinical Hemorheology 1: 85–91, 1982.

13. Bommer W, Miller L: Real-time two-dimensional color-flow Doppler: Enhanced Doppler flow imaging in the diagnosis of cardiovascular disease. Am J Cardiol 49: 944, 1982.

14. Namekawa K, Kasai C, Tsukamoto M, Koyano A: Imaging of blood flow using autocorrelation. Ultrasound in Medicine & Biology 8: 138, 1982.

15. Sahn DJ: Real-time two-dimensional Doppler echocardiographic flow mapping. Circulation 71: 849–853, 1985.

16. Ishida T, Kyo S, Motoyama T: Observation of the intracardiac blood flow in fetus by color flow mapping Doppler echocardiography. Proceedings of JSUM 45: 305–306, 1984.

17. Perry LW, Ruckman RN, Galioto FM Jr, Shapiro SR, Potter BM, Scott LP III: Echocardiographically assisted balloon atrial septostomy. Pediatrics 70: 403–408, 1982.

18. Glenn WWL, Baue AE, Geha AS, Hammond GL, Laks H: Thoracic and cardiovascular surgery, pp. 732–44. Norwalk, CT: Appleton-Century-Crofts, 1975.

19. Nadas AS, Tyler DC: Pediatric cardiology, pp. 405–26. Philadelphia: Saunders, 1972.

20. Glenn WWL, Baue AE, Geha AS, Hammond GL, Laks H: Thoracic and cardiovascular surgery, pp. 745–56. Norwalk, CT: Appleton-Century-Crofts, 1975.

21. Kyo S, Omoto R, Takamoto S, Yokote Y: Noninvasive analysis of bi-directional multi-phasic intracardiac shunts by real-time two-dimensional Doppler Echocardiography. Circulation 70 (Suppl II): II–365, 1984.

Color-coded Doppler flow imaging: a major advance for non-invasive cardiology?

J. Roelandt, W.B. Vletter, H. Rijsterborgh and W.J. Gussenhoven

Echocardiography has profoundly changed the practice of cardiology. Its diagnostic superiority results from its capacity to differentiate cardiac structures from blood-filled cavities without using contrast material. However, no direct information on blood flow is obtained and the hemodynamic consequences of minimal structural and functional abnormalities cannot be assessed. This is most apparent for lesions, such as valvular insufficiency and intracardiac shunts, which cannot be diagnosed by echocardiography alone with confidence.

After a peripheral venous injection of saline or other physiologic solutions, a bolus of blood briefly becomes 'echogenic' and echocardiography offers the possibility of studying its flow through the right heart [1]. Right-to-left shunts and tricuspid insufficiency are readily diagnosed in this manner but resolution is often less than optimal. However, the major limitation remains: no meaningful opacification of blood in the left ventricle is possible.

With the introduction of quantitative pulsed and later continuous wave Doppler echocardiography, the study of the velocity and other characteristics of intracardiac blood flow became possible [2]. Information on blood flow is obtained from a selected area or along a one-dimensional path of the ultrasound beam. When Doppler systems are integrated within the ultrasound imaging system, cross-sectional views and thus anatomical landmarks are used as background orientation for Doppler interrogation. Some systems use the audio signal for orienting the Doppler examination. Obviously, these approaches require extensive experience and operator skill. The major problem is that blood flow abnormalities are often confined to relatively small areas and require a time-consuming examination of multiple cross-sectional views using multiple sample volume positions and beam directions within each of these cross-sections. Inter-related data on structure, function, and blood flow are obtained sequentially which often makes interpretation difficult. Not the least of all problems is that spectral outputs of Doppler determined velocities are difficult to comprehend certainly by the non-expert.

Color-coded Doppler flow imaging overcomes most of these limitations. It allows real-time visualization of both spatially correlated intracardiac blood flow velocities and dispersion and superimposes them on cross-sectional images using color-coded flow schemes (Figure 1). Japanese investigators working at the Aloka and Toshiba companies pioneered most of the research and development for the production of commercially available color-coded Doppler flow imaging systems [3–5]. Independently, Bommer in the United States has designed a prototype instrument but clinical evaluation thusfar has been limited [6]. In the commercially available Japanese systems flow towards the transducer is coded as red whereas blue designates flow away from the transducer. In American proto-type instruments flow coming towards the transducer is coded in blue and flow going away from the transducer in red (in astronomy where color shifts were recognized by Christian Doppler, a red shifted star is moving away). The velocity is coded proportional to the brightness of each color. Additional parameters such as the power or amplitude intensity of the returning signals can also be displayed in one of these colors. Variance or turbulence is calculated and coded as the amount of green and yellow mixed with red or blue resulting in a mosaic pattern of colors. The color-coded blood flow data sampled at any sound beam pathway within a cardiac cross-section can also be superimposed on M-mode echocardio-grams. In a given area, at different phases in the cardiac cycle, this provides a higher temporal resolution and a wider range of velocities displayed in color, and thus provide the capability of an accurate analysis of timing and direction of blood flow. The two-dimensional flow images and M-mode flow can be shown together on the output screen or in combination with other echocardiographic information making a variety of displays available. Conventional pulsed and continuous wave Doppler spectral outputs can be selected from user designated positions within the cross-sections for accurate measurements of high velocities. Thus, color-coded Doppler flow imaging permits a comprehensive study of the direction,

⟶

Figure 1. Color-coded Doppler flow imaging of a normal heart. Apical long axis views during systole (at left) and during diastole (at right) are shown. During systole blood flow in the left ventricular cavity is away from the transducer and encoded in blue. Note the increasing brightness indicating an increasing velocity in the left ventricular outflow tract until the color changes into red. This is a result of the aliasing phenomenon when the velocity exceeds the Nyquist limit. Left ventricular inflow during diastole is encoded in red.

Figure 2. Apical long axis view of a patient with both mitral stenosis and aortic regurgitation. The frame is recorded in mid-diastole and shows the separate jets in the left ventricular cavity resulting from the stenotic mitral valve stenosis and aortic regurgitation. The mosaic of colors indicates turbulence and the velocity exceeds the limit for color display so that the color is reversed (aliasing) and the mitral jet is represented mainly in blue. Several color inversions have occured in the high-velocity jet of aortic regurgitation. Measuring the velocity in the jet would require their sampling by continuous wave Doppler.

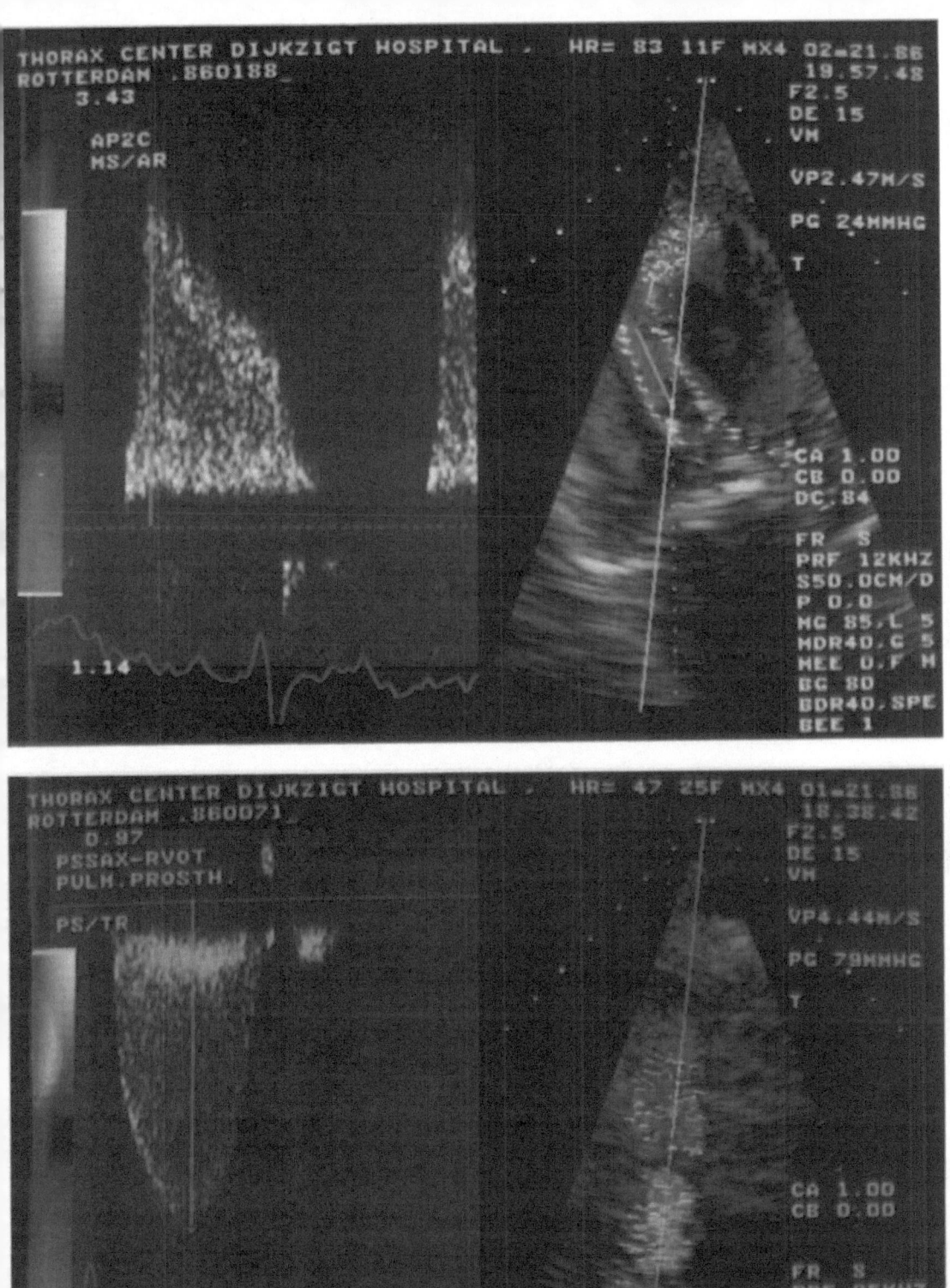

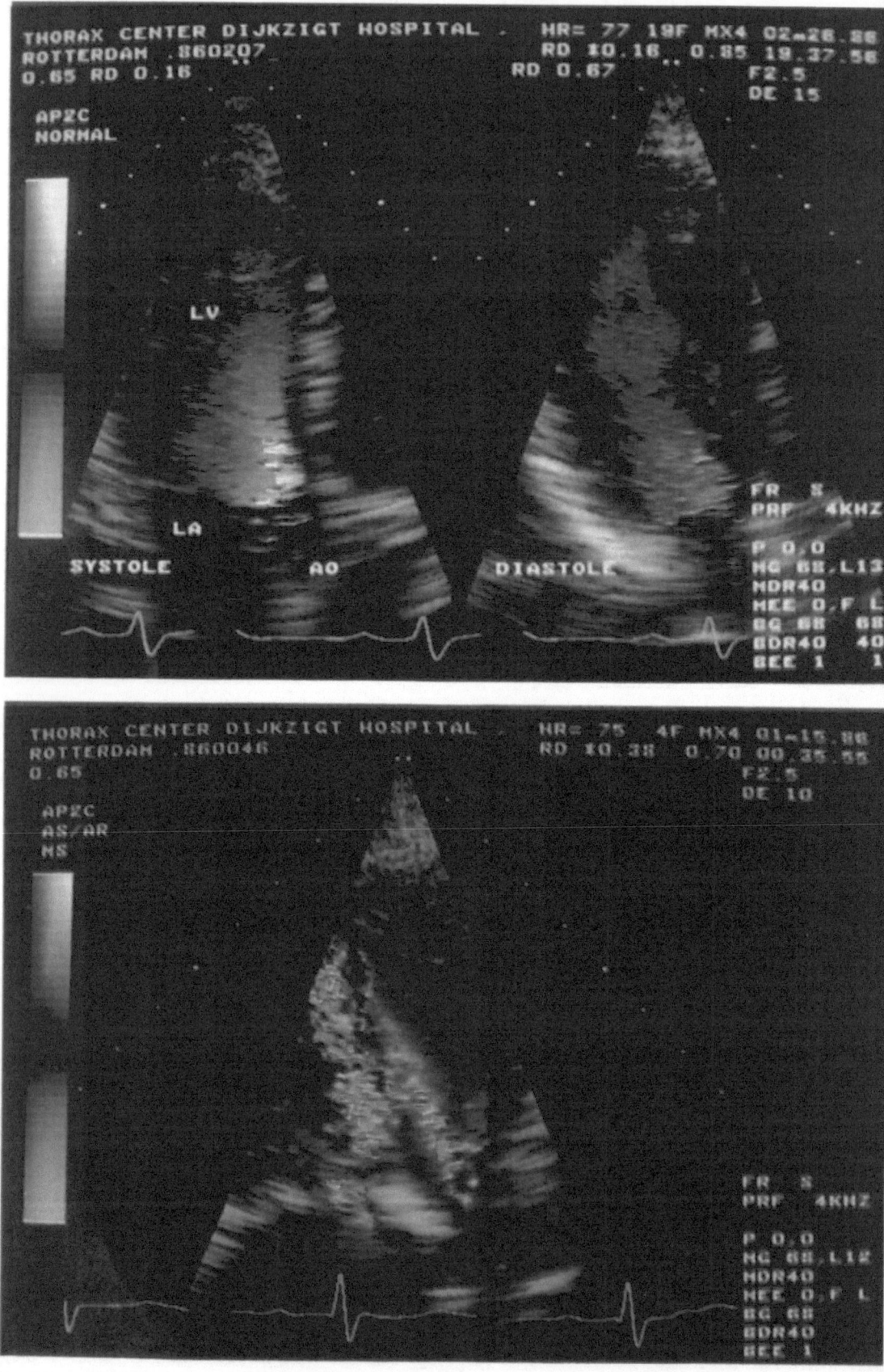

velocity, uniformity and timing of intracardiac blood flow simultaneously with an analysis of cardiac structure and function.

Color-coded Doppler flow imaging systems are based on the moving target indicator (MTI), originally developed for radar systems and autocorrelation techniques [7, 8]. Contrary to the cross-sectional imaging systems, where the echo amplitudes along a line of the sector are assembled and displayed, flow mapping systems sample the velocities of echoes along the line of sight. The MTI principle thus implies that no velocity information can be obtained from one transmit-receive cycle only. Therefore, the same line of the sector has to be addressed a number of times. This limits the highest velocities which can be measured, and/or decreases the segment size of the sector image displayed with blood flow information.

The frame rate is always lower than that of two-dimensional imaging alone as there is an inherent tradeoff between the number of successive pulses, the line density per sector scan and depth. This may cause problems in patients with very rapid heart rates such as infants and small children.

Although the technique found its origin in multigated Doppler systems [8, 9] where serial processing of blood flow information is performed at a number of discrete positions along the line of sight, the MTI blood flow velocity information is continuous, and the discrete steps (pixels) on the output screen of an MTI Doppler flow imaging system result from the speed with which analog signals are digitized in the scan converter. Aliasing which limits the maximum velocity which can be measured with pulsed Doppler systems occurs in the color-coded Doppler flow imaging systems for the same physical reasons. Aliasing indicates the ambiguous display of flow velocities which have exceeded the Nyquist limit as going in the opposite direction (the Nyquist limit is due to a sampling phenomenon which

←

Figure 3. A diastolic apical long axis view of a patient with mitral stenosis is shown to the right. The stenotic jet is visualized and bends off towards the apex as it hits the left ventricular wall. Central aliasing of high velocities in the middle of the stenotic jet which are encoded in blue create a 'flame-shaped' appearance of the jet. Continuous wave Doppler sampling is performed along a sound beam indicated on the flow map and the spectral velocity output is shown to the left. The angle between the jet flow and sound beam can be adjusted on the flow map allowing an accurate calculation of blood flow velocity. As an example the velocity has been measured at early diastole (indicated by the cursor on the spectral velocity output) and automatically calculated by machine software. The peak velocity (VP) in this beat is $2.47 \text{ m} \cdot \text{s}^{-1}$ representing a pressure difference of 24 mmHg at that particular moment in diastole.

Figure 4. A parasternal short-axis view during systole of a patient with a stenotic pulmonary Hancock prosthesis. The level of the stenotic valve is seen on the color flow map to the right. Note the increasing velocity proximal to the valve and the mosaic of colors behind it indicating a turbulent jet. The spectral output on the left was obtained by continuous wave Doppler sampling along the sound beam axis indicated on the flow map. From this recording a peak systolic velocity of $4.44 \text{ m} \cdot \text{s}^{-1}$ was calculated corresponding to a peak pressure difference across the stenotic valve of 97 mmHg.

limits the maximum frequency or velocity shift measurement to one half of the frequency at which the pulsed wave transducer transmits pulses). Thus velocities exceeding the Nyquist limit for a given pulse repetition frequency are encoded with the reversed color which gives an artifactual impression of flow reversal on the display.

Clinical uses (Table 1)

Color-coded Doppler flow imaging provides an important way to study the physiology and pathophysiology of intracardiac blood flow. Many cardiac conditions will be more easily diagnosed with the dynamic color Doppler flow maps. The spatially oriented blood flow information allows the rapid screening for abnormal blood flow patterns. This offers advantages for the diagnosis of multivalvular heart disease where the clinical differentiation may be difficult and conventional pulsed Doppler findings confusing. Examples are tricuspid regurgitation in the presence of left-sided valve disease and mixed mitral stenosis and aortic insufficiency (Figure 2). In conditions where two jetflows overlap one lesion may be overestimated or the second may be missed. Furthermore, eccentrically directed jets which are difficult to assess with conventional pulsed Doppler are now directly appreciated.

In addition to the structural abnormalities, complicated but specific flow disturbances most often characterize congenital heart diseases. Color-coded Doppler flow imaging allows a comprehensive diagnosis in most patients [10–13]. In general, more complex lesions have more lesion-specific blood flow patterns which will be more readily detected.

Aliasing gives a (multi)layered appearance to high-velocity jets with the highest velocities in the middle. In fact, in practice the aliasing phenomenon is very helpfull as it indicates in a jet the maximum velocities and their accurate direc-

Table 1. Uses of color-coded Doppler flow imaging.

1. Physiology and pathophysiology of intracardiac blood flow (velocity, turbulence, flow profile?, flow area?).
2. Rapid detection and localization of single and multiple flow abnormalities.
3. Visualization of flow jets which are difficult to find with conventional Doppler modalities (multiple shunts).
4. Determination of the spatial orientation of flow jets permits for accurate angle correction and allows a more accurate quantitative velocity measurement by continuous or pulsed wave Doppler.
5. Visualization of transvalvular and intracavitary blood flow patterns in normal and dysfunctioning prosthetic valves.
6. Semi-quantitative grading of the severity of valvular insufficiency from extent and area of regurgitant jets.

tion. Thus, these systems are helpfull in accurately measuring the maximum velocity across a stenotic or leaking valve for calculation of the pressure gradient, an application which largely stimulated the recent interest in Doppler echocardiography. Indeed the integration of continuous wave Doppler capabilities permit the guided interrogation of such high velocity jets with optimal alignment of the jet flow and sound beam or allows the accurate determination of the angle between the two (Figures 3 and 4) [14, 15]. It should be realized that a thickened calcified or prosthetic valve reflects most of the ultrasonic energy which hampers visualization of jets behind them.

One of the greatest advantages of the technique for valvular heart disease is that it facilitates the diagnosis of multivalvular disease and helps in grading of the severity of each lesion independently. Another major asset is the immediate visualization of jets which are difficult to find with conventional pulsed Doppler technique such as the presence and localization of unsuspected small septal defects or multiple defects particularly of the interventricular septum [16, 17]. Unlike large defects where velocities are low and flow is laminar smaller defects will cause jets with a turbulent high velocity. Large defects are therefore better suited to two-dimensional imaging and smaller defects for Doppler study. Direction of flow within the ventricular septal defect is of clinical importance and is better detected by color-coded Doppler flow imaging than conventional Doppler techniques [18]. This results from the fact that with pulsed Doppler, flow velocity is measured at a fixed point in the heart and the sample volume may be on different sides of the defect as a result of cardiac motion. With color-coded Doppler flow imaging the flow information is displayed upon structure and directional information is therefore more accurate. Another example where the direct reference of flow to anatomic structure is of importance is the differentiation between central and paravalvular insufficiency in patients with valve prosthesis (Figure 5). In general, flow patterns of prosthetic valve insufficiency are often eccentric and thus readily diagnosed.

With conventional Doppler systems, regurgitant lesions are diagnosed by demonstrating systolic (atrioventricular) or diastolic (semilunar) retrograde flow adjacent to the valve. Their severity is graded by measuring the extent and area of the regurgitant flow by a 'mapping technique' where a range-gated sample volume is moved around the receiving cavity. This approach is a blind technique and therefore cumbersome and time-consuming. More importantly regurgitant jets may be eccentric especially with mitral valve prolapse or leaking valve prosthesis and part of it is easily missed. The sample volume may also overlap in a contiguous chamber and detect potentially misleading flows such as e.g. in the aorta when one searches for an eccentric regurgitant jet in the left atrium.

Color Doppler allows the immediate two-dimensional visualization of flow that is in a direction opposite to what is expected at a given point in the cardiac cycle. The method therefore greatly facilitates the diagnosis of valvular insufficiency [19] (Figures 2, 6–11).

In animals with experimentally produced aortic insufficiency, the spatial distribution of the regurgitant jet was shown to be quantitatively related to the regurgitant fraction [20]. A good agreement between the planimetered surface area of the regurgitant jet and the cine-angiographic assessment of severity of mitral incompetence has been reported by Omoto et al. [21], Kitabatake et al. [22], and Miyatake et al. [23] while others have found a poor correlation [24].

Apart from experience in using the technique there are several reasons to explain this discrepancy. First, color Doppler and cineangiography usually produce different assessments of the same regurgitant jet because they present different data: the former a topographic display of velocities (first derivative of flow) and the latter a densitogram (flow distribution) of radiopaque contrast medium.

Second, there are several determinants of the length and area of a regurgitant jet (Table 2). The size and shape of the defect, the magnitude of the pressure drop* across the valve defect, and variations in compliance of the receiving chamber influence both the magnitude of the jet and its time course. An important factor in a given patient is the anatomic shape of the valvular defect. Irregularities of the defect will cause turbulence leading to a loss of kinetic energy. With increasing turbulence the length/area of the jet will decrease while the regurgitant volume and its distribution can be quite the same.

It must further be realized that a small regurgitant volume may cause severe symptoms when atrial compliance is low as pressure in the left atrium steeply

---

* The word gradient is commonly misused in cardiology. A gradient in blood flow indicates how steeply a pressure varies with distance and it is this variation which produces its acceleration. Thus a pressure gradient does not indicate a pressure difference or drop.

Table 2. Determinants of length and area of regurgitant jets on color-coded Doppler flow images.

1. Size of defect.
2. Pressure difference across the defect ($\triangle P$).
3. Pressure difference as a function of time (slope $\triangle P_t$) (influenced by regurgitant volume and compliance of receiving chamber).
4. Shape of the defect (may induce turbulence which causes losses in kinetic energy).

$\longrightarrow$

Figure 5. An apical view and systolic color flow map of a patient with a Hancock prosthesis. Two systolic regurgitant jets are seen in the right atrium representing a central and paravalvular leak.

Figure 6. Color Doppler flow map of a patient with subvalvular aortic stenosis. During systole (left panel) the level of the discrete membranous obstruction in the outflow tract is seen with the jet of mosaic colors indicating turbulence behind it. Note the increasing velocity proximal to the obstruction resulting in aliasing. During diastole (right panel) the high velocity jet of aortic regurgitation strikes the anterior mitral leaflet and then reaches the apex.

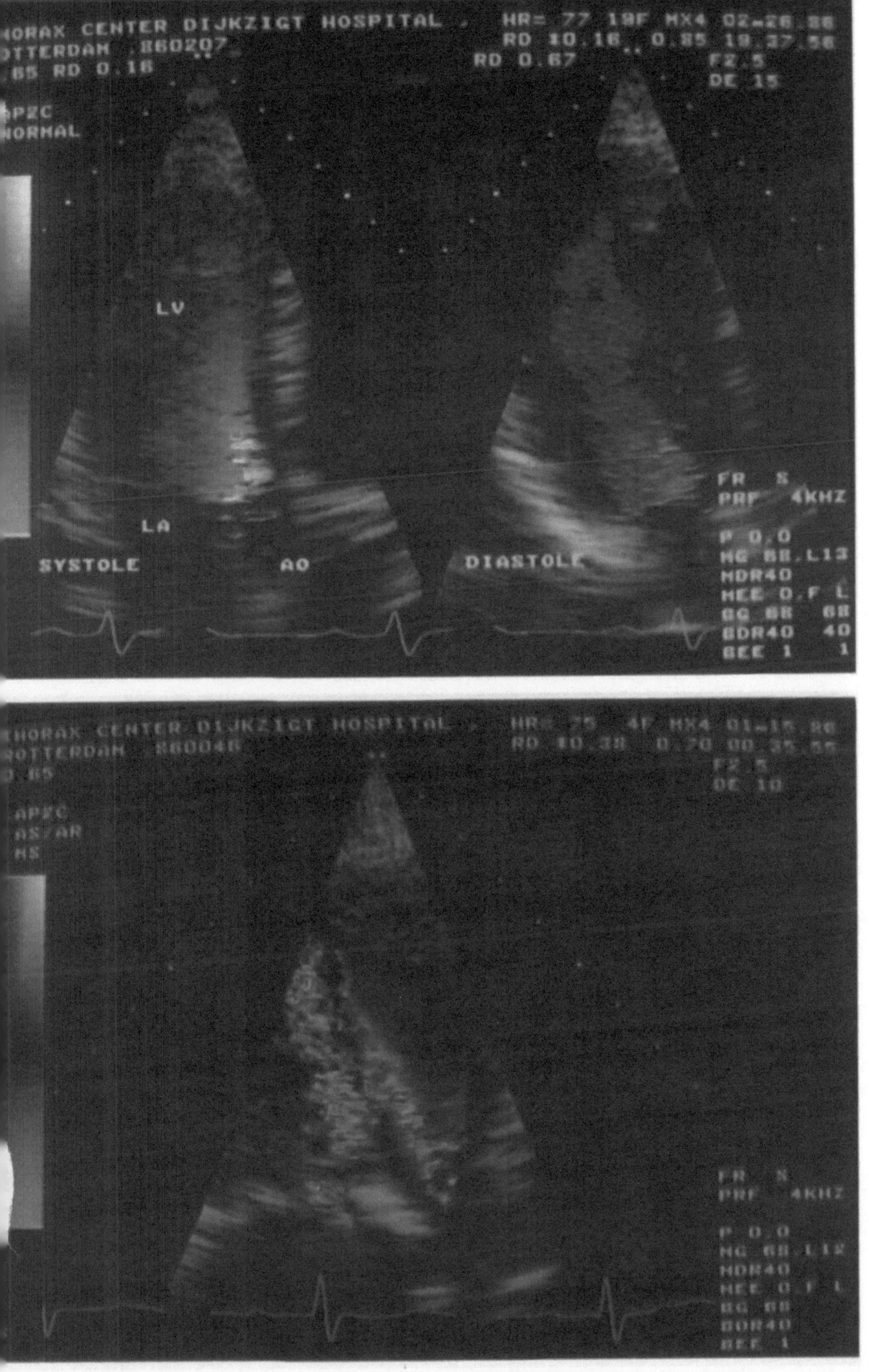

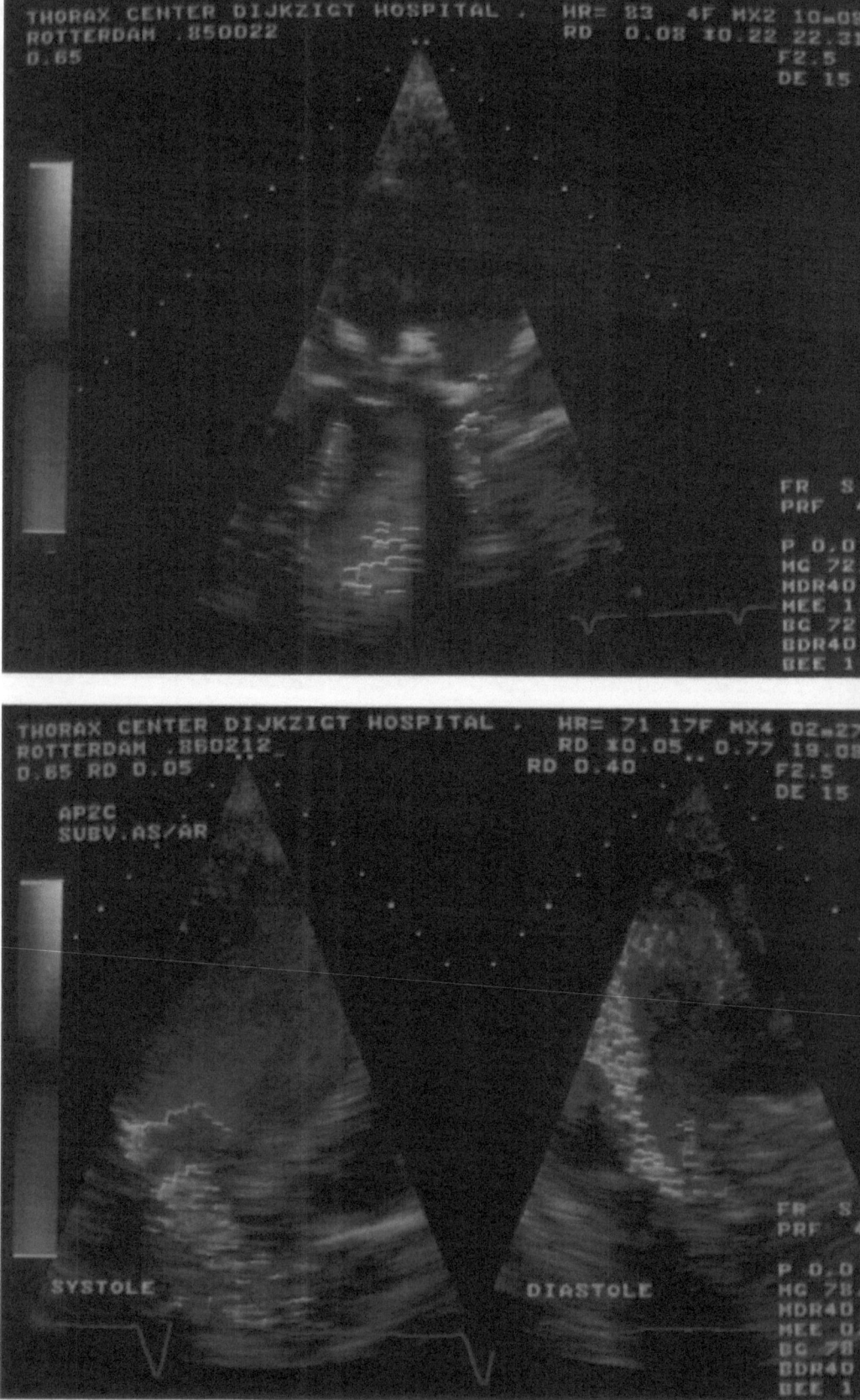

SYSTOLE   DIASTOLE

increases (Figure 12). Thus for clinical decision-making the Doppler imaging-defined information is but one of the many factors to be considered in the assessment of a patient with mitral regurgitation.

Third, there are inherent problems related to the Doppler technique. Velocity measurements are dependent upon the alignment of the jet flow and sound beam. If this angle increases from one area to another within the jet, the velocities measured in a certain area may be too low to be coded, since the machine has a lower velocity threshold. Future instruments should incorporate an automatic angle correction before color coding, but currently the lower velocities at the perimeter of the regurgitant jet and more particularly at its tail may fall below the threshold for color-coding. As a result the degree of insufficiency will be underestimated. This may be important when evaluating tricuspid insufficiency where velocities are often low. A solution to this problem may be the power spectrum display, a feature of the Toshiba SSH65A system, which theoretically allows a velocity as low as 3 cm/s to be encoded. Clinical evaluation of this feature is in progress [25].

There are other technical factors which may affect the color coding. The signal-to-noise ratio by influencing gain settings have an effect on the display of the surface area of a jet and so do the MTI filter characteristics which separate blood flow velocity shifts from velocity shifts introduced by anatomical structures and/or reverberations (clutter). The higher the order of the filter, the more effectively 'non-flow' information is suppressed and the less is the effect of the gain settings.

Thus despite great and widespread enthusiasm, quantification of regurgitant lesions can only be semi-quantitative at best and a close agreement with angiocardiography would not be expected in the individual patient.

Although not yet widely used clinically, another application of Doppler echocardiography is the measurement of volume flow and cardiac output. The major limitation lies in the accuracy of the measurement of cross-sectional flow area rather than the velocity measurement (mean temporal velocity times area of flow yields volume flow). Theoretically the 'area of flow' would be a more accurate measurement than the anatomical area and can be directly obtained from color flow images. Hoit et al. [26] reported good agreement between color Doppler

---

Figure 7. Systolic apical long axis views of a patient with mitral regurgitation. Color-coded Doppler flow mapping in the right panel shows the jet of mitral regurgitation with a mosaic of colors indicating turbulence. Blood flow in the outflow tract demonstrates increasing velocity and aliasing. The patient had mild symptomatic mitral regurgitation.

Figure 8. Apical long axis view of a patient with prolapse of the anterior mitral valve leaflet. The regurgitant jet is eccentric and is directed towards the lateral left atrial wall. Note the mosaic pattern which indicates the turbulence and the increasing blood velocity proximal to the defect within the left ventricular cavity. Note that conventional blind Doppler interrogation may result in recording the velocity within the ventricle and the presence of the eccentric jet may have been missed.

derived areas of flow and calculated flow areas from cardiac output and conventional Doppler time velocity integrals in experimental animals. Valdez-Cruz et al. [27] found cardiac output measurements using color Doppler derived flow areas more accurate than when anatomically derived areas of flow were used at low cardiac output states. One must realize, however, that the lower velocities at the boundaries of flow are not encoded for reasons discussed above. Furthermore, improvements on the resolution of flow imaging seem necessary in order to decrease the measurement variability which is quite high.

Thus, further clinical validation and results from other centers are needed and the application of measurement of volume flow will become a major research goal.

Color-coded Doppler flow imaging will open a new area of research as transvalvular and intracavitary flow patterns can be studied which will add to a better understanding of some clinical conditions.

Prosthetic valves have characteristic transprosthetic flow patterns and their changes may be helpful in the early diagnosis of valve dysfunction [28] (Figure 13). Maximal anterograde transprosthetic flow is readily seen and used to guide a continuous wave Doppler cursor through the maximal velocity allowing an accurate baseline pressure drop across the prosthesis. In patients with a Hancock bioprosthesis in the mitral position investigators of the Stanford group have noted a deviation of flow towards the septum reversing the direction of normal intraventricular flow. Such an abnormal pattern may represent a significant loss of mechanical energy in such patients and may be an important factor when left ventricular function is compromized. The method may also help us understand why some patients after a myocardial infarction have a laminated thrombus while others develop a pedunculated thrombus carrying a much higher risk for systemic embolization [29].

→

Figure 9. Apical four chamber view of a patient with mitral valve prolapse and ruptured chordae tendinae resulting in severe symptomatic mitral regurgitation. Note the wide area and extent of turbulent flow in the left atrium confirming severe mitral regurgitation. A single Doppler line is selected and indicated on the flow map. The blood flow velocity and its dispersion at each point along this interrogating Doppler beam axis is displayed in color superimposed on the M-mode echocardiogram (at left). In addition to a better temporal resolution for studying time relationships a wider range of velocity is now displayed more particularly in the low velocity range.

Figure 10. A parasternal short axis view at aortic valve level shows severe tricuspid regurgitation indicated by the wide area of turbulent flow (demonstrated by the mosaic of colors). Velocity of the regurgitant jet allows estimation of right ventricular systolic pressure and hence pulmonary artery pressure. Continuous wave Doppler sampling is performed along the sound beam axis shown on the flow map. The spectral velocity output is shown on the left and peak systolic velocity (VP) is $2.93 \, m \cdot s^{-1}$ corresponding to a peak systolic pressure difference of 34 mmHg between the right ventricle and right atrium. Adding clinically estimated central venous pressure provides an estimated right ventricular systolic pressure of 45 mmHg.

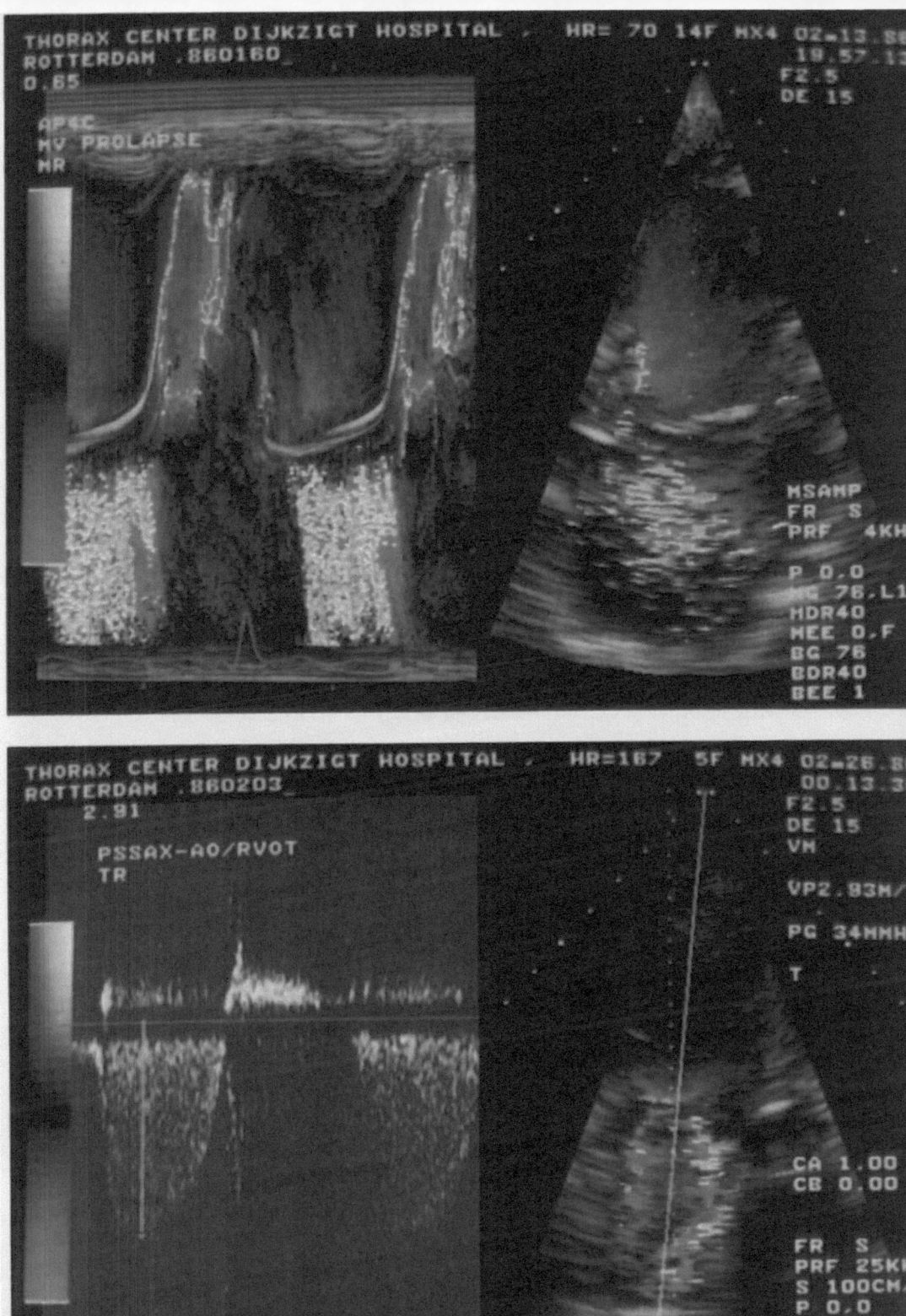

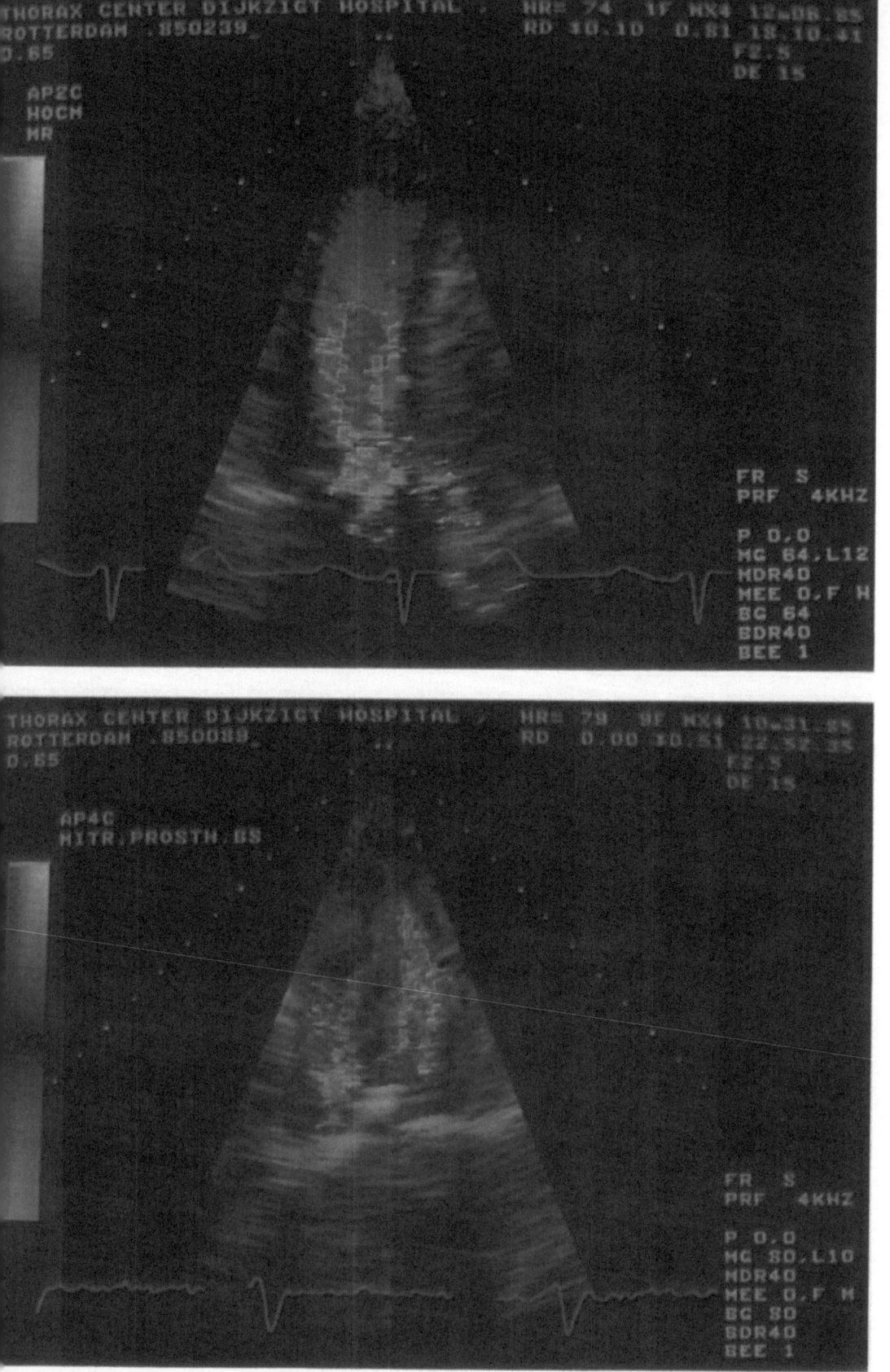

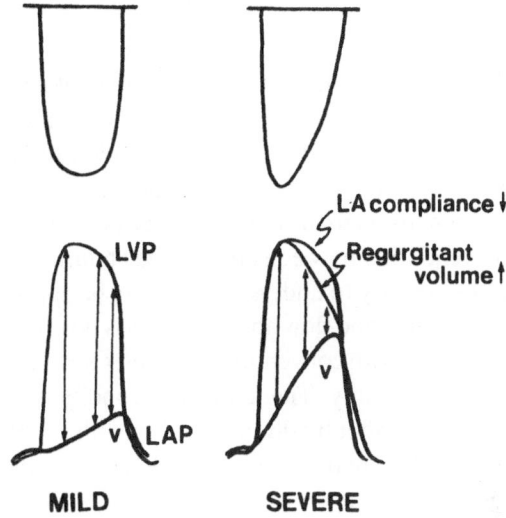

Figure 12. Doppler flow patterns in mitral insufficiency. In mild mitral regurgitation when there is a small regurgitant volume there is a sustained high systolic pressure in the left ventricle (LVP). The pressure in the moderate increase in left atrial pressure (LAP) causes a small V-wave. As a result, the pressure difference between left ventricle and left atrium will remain high throughout systole resulting in a sustained high regurgitant velocity. In severe symptomatic mitral regurgitation, when the regurgitant volume is large, the pressure in the left ventricle will rapidly decrease while the pressure in the left atrium increases resulting in a high V-wave. At the end of systole the pressure difference between ventricle and left atrium will be low, resulting in a low regurgitant velocity. When left atrial compliance is low as in acute regurgitation the regurgitant volume is relatively low. In these circumstances pressure in the left atrium will rapidly increase resulting in a similar pattern.

Intraoperative color-coded Doppler flow imaging has been used to verify the preoperative diagnosis and to help surgical decision-making [30, 31]. The method further allows the result of valve replacement and intracardiac repair to be assessed before chest closure.

←

Figure 11. Apical long axis view and color-coded flow map of a patient with hypertrophic obstructive cardiomyopathy. The frame is selected in mid-systole and shows increasing velocity towards the outflow tract with a turbulent flow in the subaortic area. Two turbulent jets are seen as a mosaic of colors – one which is obliquely oriented towards the anterior aortic valve and the other one indicates the mitral regurgitation.

Figure 13. Apical long axis view obtained from a patient with a mitral Björk Shiley prosthetic valve. Transprosthetic blood flow is seen as two jets originating from the major and minor orifices. Velocity in the middle of the jets exceeds the set limits for color display resulting in central aliasing.

Conclusion

Conventional Doppler techniques are limited to sampling one specific cardiac site at a time. Color-coded Doppler flow imaging provides a spatially oriented display of intracardiac blood flow and permits information to be appreciated which is meaningless in the absence of a spatial reference. This 'ultrasonic angiocardiography' adds a new dimension to the ultrasonic analysis of the heart since it allows the immediate differentiation between normal and abnormal blood flow. The abnormal flow patterns are easy to understand and can be appreciated by non-experts. Quicker screening for blood flow abnormalities is possible and the abnormalities we presently diagnose with conventional Doppler techniques are diagnosed with a greater degree of certainty. The number of conditions which we can diagnose with confidence will undoubtedly increase and the pathophysiology of some clinical conditions will be better understood. We believe that most, if not all of the applications of pulsed Doppler echocardiography will be replaced by this new technique. It will be used in combination with continuous wave Doppler for sampling high velocity areas. Both techniques will be used interactively just like two-dimensional and M-mode echocardiography which provides high temporal resolution information from selected areas within the cross-sectional image.

Acknowledgement

We thank Toshiba Medical Systems Europe for providing the SSH65A instrument for clinical evaluation and Tineke van der Kolk for her secretarial help.

References

1. Roelandt J: Contrast echocardiography. Ultrasound Med & Biol 8: 471–92, 1982.
2. Hatle L, Angelsen B: Doppler ultrasound in cardiology (2nd ed). Philadelphia: Lea & Febiger, 1985.
3. Namekawa K, Kasai C, Tsukamato M, Koyano A: Imaging of blood flow using autocorrelation. Ultrasound in Med & Biol 8: 132 (Abstract), 1982.
4. Omoto R, Yokote Y, Takamoto S et al.: Clinical significance of newly developed real-time intracardiac two-dimensional blood flow imaging system (2-D Doppler). Jpn Circ J 47: 974 (Abstract), 1983.
5. Iimuma K, Seo Y, Skirasaka T, Hongo H, Sasaki H: Real-time two-dimensional ultrasound blood flow imaging system. J Ultrasound Med 2: 66 (Abstract), 1983.
6. Bommer WJ, Miller L: Real-time two-dimensional color-flow Doppler. Enhanced Doppler flow imaging in the diagnosis of cardiovascular disease. Am J Cardiol 49: 944 (Abstract), 1982.
7. Nowicki A, Reid JH: An infinite gate pulse Doppler. Ultrasound in Med & Biol 7: 41–50, 1981.
8. Brandestini MA. Topoflow: a digital full range Doppler velocitymeter. IEEE Son-Ultrason SU25-5: 287–93, 1978.
9. Brandestini MA, Eyer MK, Stevenson JG: M/Q mode echocardiography – the synthesis of

conventional echo with digital multigate Doppler. In : Lancée CT(ed.) Proc. 3rd Symposium Echocardiology, pp. 207–12. The Hague, Boston, London: Martinus Nijhoff Publishers, 1979.

10. Omoto R, Kasai C, Namekawa K et al.: Real-time two-dimensional Doppler echocardiography. Tokyo: Shindan-To-Chiryo Co, 1983.

11. Yanagisawa M, Yano S, Shiraishi H, Nakajima Y, Kuramatsu T, Itoh K, Suzuki O: Application of two-dimensional Doppler echocardiography to the diagnosis of congenital heart diseases in infancy. J Cardiovasc Ultrasonography 3: 317–24, 1984.

12. Kyo S, Omoto R, Takamoto S, Takanawa E: Clinical significance of color flow mapping real-time two-dimensional Doppler echocardiography (2-D Doppler) in congenital heart disease. Circulation 70 (Suppl. II): II–37 (Abstract), 1984.

13. Suzuki Y, Kambara H, Kadota K, Tamaki S, Yamazato A, Nohara R, Osakada G, Kawai C: Detection of intracardiac shunt flow in atrial septal defect using a real-time two-dimensional color-coded Doppler flow imaging system and comparison with contrast two-dimensional echocardiography. Am J Cardiol 56: 347–350, 1985.

14. Sahn DH, Valdes Cruz LM, Swensson RE, Scagnelli S, Dalton N: Potential for angular errors in Doppler gradient estimates: a study of spatial orientation of jet lesions using real-time color flow Doppler imaging. Circulation 70 (Suppl. II): II–115 (Abstract), 1984.

15. Nakagawa H, Miyatake K, Izumi S, Kinoskita N, Sakakibara H, Nimura Y: Application of real-time two-dimensional Doppler flow imaging system for the measurement of pressure gradient across the mitral valve in mitral stenosis. J Am Coll Cardiol 5: 403 (Abstract), 1985.

16. Sahn DJ, Swensson RE, Valdes Cruz LM, Scagnelli S, Main J: Two-dimensional color flow mapping for evaluation of ventricular septal defect shunts: a new diagnostic modality. Circulation 70 (supp. II): II–364 (Abstract), 1984.

17. Ortiz E, Robinson PJ, Deanfield JE, Franklin R, Macartney FJ, Wyse RKH: Localization of ventricular septal defects by simultaneous display of superimposed colour Doppler and cross sectional echocardiographic images. Br Heart J 54: 53–60, 1985.

18. Stevenson JG, Kawabori I, Brandestini MA: Color coded visualization of flow within ventricular septal defects: implications for peak pulmonary artery pressure. Am J Cardiol 49: 911, 1982.

19. Miyataka K, Okamoto M, Kinoshita N et al.: Clinical applications of a new type of real-time two-dimensional flow imaging system. Am J Cardiol 54: 857–68, 1984.

20. Sahn DJ, Valdes-Cruz L, Scagnelli S, Tomizuka F, Elias W, Covell J: Two-dimensional Doppler color flow mapping for spatial localization and quantification of aortic insufficiency: validation of a new diagnostic modality using an open chest animal model. Circulation 70 (supp. II): II–38 (Abstract), 1984.

21. Omoto R, Yokote Y, Takamoto S, Kyo S, Ueda K, Asano H, Namekawa K, Kasai C, Kondo Y, Koyano A: The development of real-time two-dimensional Doppler echocardiography and its clinical significance in acquired valvular diseases: with specific reference to the evaluation of valvular regurgitation. Jpn Heart J 25: 325, 1984.

22. Kitabatake A, Masuyama T, Asao M, Tanouchi J, Morita T, Ito H, Hori M, Inoue M, Abe H: Noninvasive estimation of the degree of regurgitation from two-dimensional (2-D) Doppler-Echo (flow stucture) cardiac image. Circulation 68 (suppl. III): III–367 (Abstract), 1983.

23. Miyatake K, Izumi S, Okamoto M et al.: Semiquantitative grading of severity of mitral regurgitation by real-time two-dimensional Doppler flow imaging technique. J Am Coll Cardiol 7: 82–8, 1986.

24. Yock PG, Segal J, Teirstein PS, Schnittger I, Popp R: Doppler color flow mapping: utility in valvular regurgitation. Circulation 70 (suppl. II): II–38 (Abstract), 1984.

25. Machii K, Hirai H, Nishizawa S et al.: Left ventricular flow pattern in myocardial infarction assessed by power-mode two-dimensional color flow mapping. J Am Coll Cardiol 7: 135 (Abstract), 1986.

26. Hoit B, Bhargava V, Swensson R, Sattn D: Determination of flow area in echo Doppler calculations of cardiac output: investigation of flow orifices using real-time, two-dimensional

echo Doppler color flow mapping. Circulation 70 (suppl. II): II–39 (Abstract), 1984.

27. Valdez-Cruz L, Elias W, Dalton N, Hagan-Ansart S, Sahn D, Swensson R, Sherman F: Comparison of cardiac flows calculated with color coded Doppler flow mapping and conventional Doppler techniques: validation studies in an open chest animal model. J Am Coll Cardiol 5: 452 (Abstract), 1985.

28. Bommer W, Tam K, Ehret R, Rebeck K: Two-dimensional real-time flow mapping of prosthetic heart valves. J Am Coll Cardiol 5: 526, 1985.

29. Visser C, Kan G, Meltzer RS, Dunning AJ, Roelandt J: Embolic potential of left ventricular thrombus after myocardial infarction: a two-dimensional echocardiographic study of 119 patients. J Am Coll Cardiol 5: 1276–80 (Abstract), 1985.

30. Takamoto S, Kyo S, Adachi H, Matsumura M, Yokote Y, Omoto R: Intraoperative color flow mapping by real-time two-dimensional Doppler echocardiography for evaluation of valvular and congenital heart disease and vascular disease. J Thorac Cardiovasc Surg 90: 802–12, 1985.

31. Dagli SV, Nanda NC, Roitman D, Moos S, Hsiung MC, Nath PH, Soto B: Evaluation of aortic dissection by Doppler color flow mapping. Am J Cardiol 56: 497–498, 1985.

III. Clinical advances in Doppler echocardiography

Impact of Doppler cardiography on clinical management in adult cardiology

Terje Skjaerpe

Introduction

With Doppler cardiography (Doppler) the velocity and direction of blood flow is measured. Consequently Doppler should be useful in diagnosing heart diseases mainly affecting these parameters. Valvular stenosis (increased velocities) and valvular regurgitation (reversed velocities) are the classical examples of such diseases.

In a broader sense, any cardiac malfunction affects the blood flow. Sometimes this effect is difficult to measure with conventional Doppler (coronary artery stenosis),but in most cardiac patients Doppler will provide important information to the doctor regarding clinical decision-making.

Research on Doppler has to a large extent concentrated on obtaining hemo-dynamic information which would otherwise require invasive investigations. When such information can be obtained by Doppler, the noninvasive nature of the method makes it a superior tool compared to catheterization in patient follow up. In addition, some information can be obtained by Doppler which is more difficult, or impossible to obtain by other methods.

In the following I will try to indicate how Doppler may help the clinician in patient management, and also how to avoid the most important pitfalls. The last point is crucial in patient care, since misinterpretation of Doppler recordings may lead to wrong decisions of serious consequence to the patient.

Valve stenosis

Doppler as a quantitative method in stenotic lesions is based on the relationship between velocity and pressure drop. This relationship is fairly complicated, involving inertia of the blood (because the flow is pulsatile), viscosity, and the force needed to accelerate blood across the obstruction (convective acceleration) [1]. The break-trough occurred when Holen and coworkers showed that in significant stenosis both inertia and viscosity is of minor importance, and that the velocity in the stenotic jet is directly related to the pressure drop across the obstruction [2]. This relationship was further simplified by Hatle *et al.* [3], resulting in the equation known as 'The simplified Bernoulli equation': *Pressure drop = 4 × Vmax²*, where Vmax is the maximal velocity in the stenotic jet. In addition to these pioneering works, several experimental and clinical studies [4–8] have confirmed the surprisingly high accuracy of this simple equation in calculating pressure drop from velocity.

In every day practice the situation is more complicated, mainly for two reasons: (a) The signal from the jet may be very weak, preventing the velocities from being displayed, and (b) the angle between the ultrasound beam and the direction of the jet may be too large, resulting in underestimation of velocity and pressure drop.

The first problem is overcome by using equipment with optimal sensitivity. This still involves the use of a separate Doppler transducer. A combined echo/ Doppler transducer will usually reduce the time spent in searching for the jet velocities, but the final recordings should always be made with the separate transducer. This is mandatory in aortic stenosis, whereas the sensitivity is less critical in stenotic lesions of the other valves. When the signal is weak, it is also useful to apply a high degree of compression and minimal reject, and to apply maximal high pass filtering to remove low frequency, high intensity components from the displayed signal.

The second problem necessitates the recording of jet velocities from multiple directions. This is again of critical importance in aortic stenosis (Fig. 1), but the procedure should always be considered in other stenotic lesions also.

The limitation of Doppler in assessing pressure drop, is that no special marker seems to indicate that the correct velocities are recorded. Potentially then, pressure drops may be underestimated. If Doppler is to be trusted in a single case, the procedure described is unavoidable. The reward is great, however, since experience shows that a small angle to the flow can be obtained in all patients, and that the pressure drop across any stenotic valve can be assessed with an accuracy comparable to that of invasive pressure recordings [3, 4–8]. Little documentation exists on tricuspid stenosis, but in those few examined at our laboratory, the invasive and noninvasive pressure drops have been close to identical. The consequense is that catheterization to a large extent is made superfluous in the preoperative follow up of patients with valve stenosis. Repeated recordings can be made as frequent as needed, providing a better base for the decision on when to operate.

Since the pressure drop not only changes with valve area, but also with flow across the valve, the pressure drop may sometimes be severely misleading in assessing the severity of the lesion (Figure 2). Assessment of valve area is therefore often necessary. Methods have been developed to achieve this either by Doppler alone [9] or by combined use of Doppler and echo [10–12] in mitral and aortic stenosis. Two of the methods [9, 11, 12] are applicable in the presence of

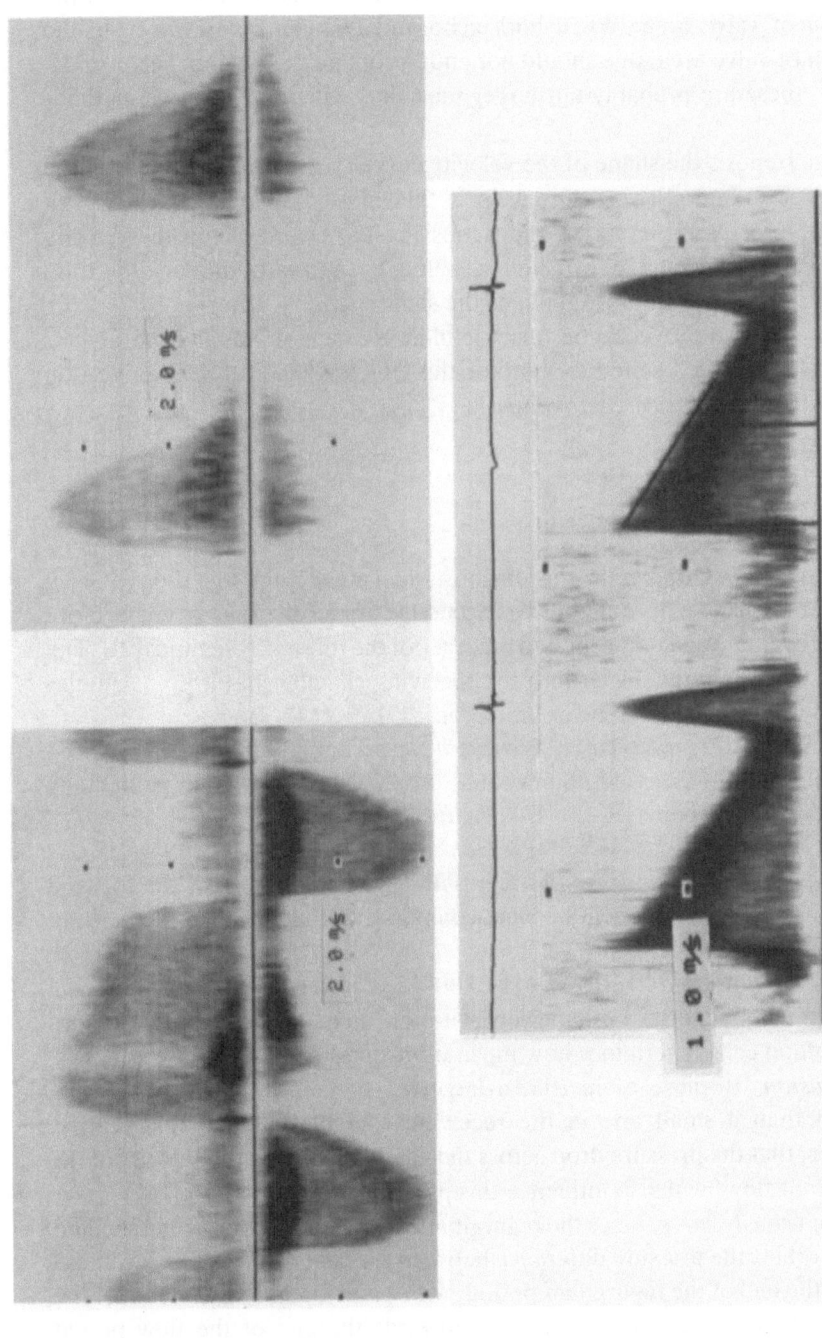

Figure 1. Velocity recordings from the stenotic jet in a patient with aortic stenosis. Left: Recording from the apex. Calculated peak pressure drop is 73 mmHg. Right: Recording from the second right intercostal space. Calculated peak pressure drop is 92 mmHg.

Figure 2. Velocity recording from a patient with mitral stenosis. Mean pressure drop was calculated to 3 mmHg. The pressure half time, indicated by the two vertical lines in the second beat, is 300 ms, giving a calculated valve area of 0.7 cm^2. The low pressure drop is explained by the slow heart rate and a low cardiac output.

combined stenosis and regurgitation, even also when both valves on the left side are leaking. In that case, in aortic stenosis, no other routine method exists for the estimation of valve area. When both echo and Doppler are involved in the estimation of valve area, one should not underestimate the potential errors [12]. However, these are probably not larger than those made by invasive methods [13].

In aortic stenosis the shape of the velocity curve give some indications on the severity in addition to the pressure drop. If the velocity curve has an early peak with a rapid decrease thereafter, the stenosis is less severe than if the velocity curve appears more rounded, with high velocities even towards the end of systole, even if the peak pressure drop remains the same.

Doppler has also proved to be very useful in assessing supra- and subvalvular stenosis [14]. It is well suited to monitor the effect of medical intervention on dynamic obstructions in the left ventricle.

Valvular regurgitation

The sensitivity of Doppler in the diagnosis of valvular regurgitations is well established [15–20]. The quantitative accuracy of the method is much more difficult to evaluate due to the limited accuracy of the reference methods [21]. The intrusion of the regurgitant jet into the receiving chamber has in some studies correlated well to angiographic examinations [17].

Limitations to this method exist, however [22]. At our laboratory we have tried to assess the effect of the regurgitant volume on several hemodynamic parameters as recorded with Doppler [18–20, 23] (Figures 3 and 4):

a *Velocity of forward flow.* As the regurgitant volume increases, the forward velocity across the valve will become comparatively higher than the velocity across sufficient valves.

b *Intensity of the Doppler signal.* The intensity of the back-scattered signal increases with increasing volume regurgitation, since, within limits, the number of blood cells determines how much ultrasound is back-scattered.

c *Jet intrusion.* Because of inertia, a large regurgitant volume is less easily stopped than a small one in the receiving chamber. One should realize, however, that the pressure drop across the valve, predicting the velocity of the regurgitant flow, will also influence this parameter.

d *Shape of velocity curve.* Since the regurgitant volume empties one chamber and fills the other, the pressure difference between the chambers tends to decrease toward the end of the regurgitant period, with a corresponding decrease of the velocity. Steeply decreasing velocities towards the end of the flow period therefore indicate a large regurgitation.

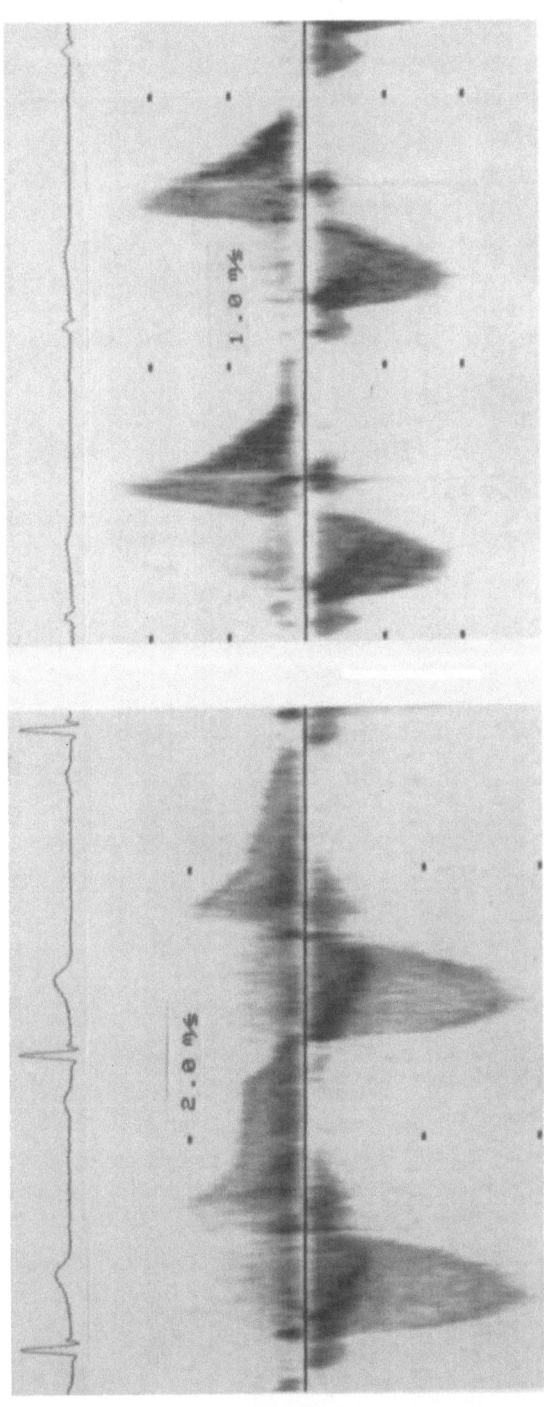

Figure 3. Velocity recordings from two patients with pulmonary stenosis, after valvulotomy. Left: Systolic peak pressure drop is 51 mmHg. The regurgitation is mild as indicated by the moderate decrease in velocities in the last part of diastole. Right: A more extensive valvulotomi as indicated by a lower peak pressure drop (10 mmHg), and a more pronounced regurgitation (steeply decreasing diastolic velocities). There is equilibration of pressures in the right ventricle and the pulmonary artery shortly after mid-diastole.

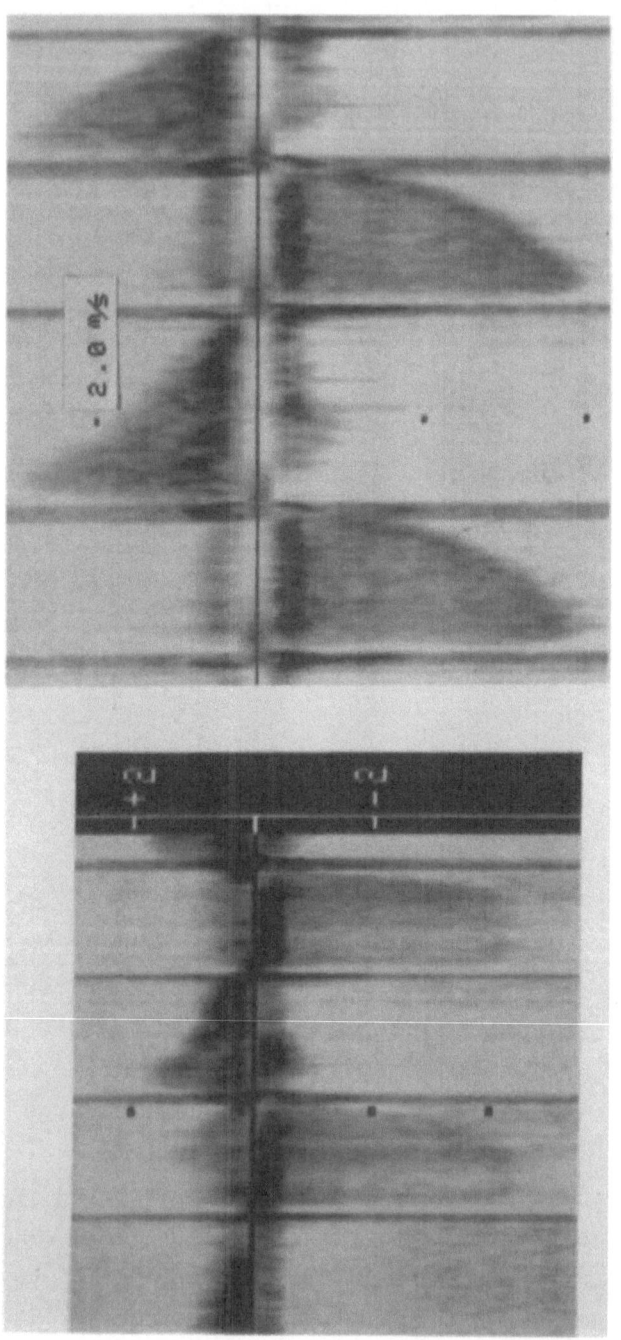

Figure 4. Left: Velocity recording through a mitral valve prosthesis two weeks after operation. A small paravalvular leak is recorded. Right: A recording made 2 months later. A much more severe regurgitation is recorded as indicated by 1) higher signal intensity, 2) significant increase in diastolic flow, and 3) steeply decreasing velocities in the regurgitant flow towards end systole because of the build-up of a large V-wave in the left atrium. There was no increase in pressure half time.

In addition, the effect of the regurgitation upon the flow in vessels proximal [24, 25] or distal [26] to the regurgitant valve, may indicate the severity.

In our opinion, none of these parameters represent the final clue to the problem, and since some are difficult to quantitate and express by figures, it is probably wise to gain some experience before the method is extensively used to decide upon patient management. By combining the information, however, a very useful estimate of the severity can be obtained, and we experience a growing need to confirm or correct the angiographic findings by Doppler.

A very interesting way to quantitate regurgitant fraction is to measure stroke volume through the insufficient valve and through a competent valve [27, 28]. The regurgitant volume can then be calculated. The limitation is given by the inaccuracy of the stroke volume estimates (see below).

Valve prosthesis

Doppler probably provides the most powerful tool available for the evaluation of prosthetic valve function. In critical ill patients a potentially harmful catheterization can be avoided. It will also reduce the time delay before reoperation.

In essence, obstructions and leaks (Figure 4) are assessed as in native valves, except that the combined use of Doppler and echocardiography is necessary to be able to decide if a leak is paravalvular or not, and where a paravalvular leak is located. One important pitfall to be aware of, is that regurgitations in mitral disk valve prosthesis may sometimes be very difficult to record from the apex. This is because the disk will be in the closed position during the regurgitant period, preventing ultrasound to penetrate into the left atrium. In such patients it may be useful to place the transducer in the left parasternal position, and place the sample volume on the atrial side of the prosthesis. Disturbed flow, caused by the regurgitation, may then be recorded. Indirect evidence of the regurgitation can be obtained by recording increased forward flow across the prosthesis compared to the flow across other valves, when there is no increase in pressure half time. If the pressure half time is prolonged, obstruction of the prosthesis is likely.

It is considered important to obtain baseline recordings shortly after surgery since the 'normal' velocities across a prosthetic valve may vary quite a lot, depending on the size of the prosthesis in relation to the patient [1].

Left ventricular performance

The cardiac output may be looked upon as a measure of global left ventricular performance. A lot of research has been done to evaluate Doppler and echocardiography as a method to quantitate volume flow. Reviewing the literature, from which I have listed some articles [29–34], it soon becomes apparent that no general agreement has been reached on how to do the measurements. If we concentrate on aortic flow, we find that flow area measurements have been made at the aortic annulus, the sinus of Valsalva and at levels distal to the sinus of Valsalva. In some presentations the level for diameter measurements is not specified. Considering the large variations in cross sectional area at these levels [35], it is surprising that all seem to give a good correlation to invasive measurements. If the blood velocity changes inversely with flow area, the results could be explained. However, that does not seem to be the case [30]. Theoretically, a flat velocity profile is most likely found at the aortic annulus [1]. We therefore recommend to measure flow area and flow velocity at this level.

The variability of diameter measurements on repeated recordings is probably in the range of 1–2 mm. The resulting error on cardiac output estimations is about 10–20%. The smallest changes in flow velocity which can be detected with Doppler, is probably about 10% [36]. Total errors of 20–30% in estimated cardiac output is therefore to be expected, even at the theoretical best opinion in the aorta. The estimates may nevertheless be quite useful to the clinician, but more important is that changes in cardiac output (changes in velocity integral) can be assessed quite accurately, since errors made by diameter measurements are excluded. The acute effects of various pacing modes and drug interventions can thus be evaluated.

The shape of the velocity curve in the aorta may give information about the left ventricular performance [37], for instance to what extent a low cardiac output is caused by myocardial failure or hypovolemia [1]. The mitral velocity curve may indicate the diastolic performance. When there is increased resistance to filling, either because of hypertrophy or because of increased diastolic pressure, it is a common observation that the velocities during the active filling phase increase, while they tend to decrease during the passive phase.

In pericardial effusion, the changes in stroke volume during respiration, giving rise to the paradoxic pulse, is easily recorded (Figure 5).

Right heart pressure estimation

Several methods have been developed to estimate the right ventricular or pulmonary artery pressure [38–44]. At our laboratory we consider the recording of the velocities in tricuspid regurgitation to provide the most accurate estimate of the systolic pressure on the right side [41–44]. It is also widely applicable because of the high frequency of tricuspid regurgitation in patients with increased pressures [42], and because of the high sensitivity of the method [19].

The isovolumetric relaxation time of the right ventricle (Pc/To interval) is useful in patients without right heart failure and significant tricuspid regurgitation [38, 41]. One possible pitfall should be mentioned. In tachycardia, or in low cardiac output states, the initial opening of the tricuspid valve can be difficult to

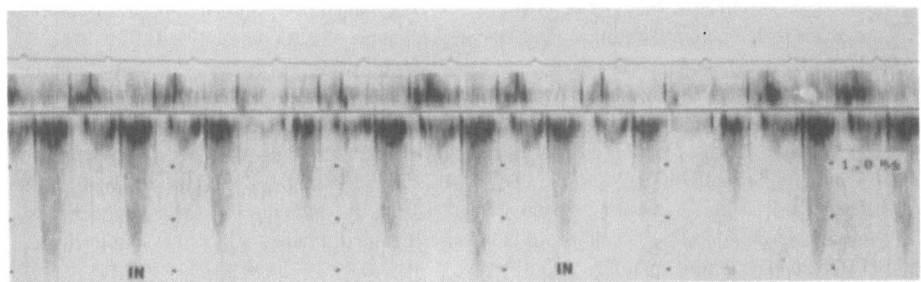

Figure 5. Velocity recording across an aortic valve prosthesis one week after operation. There is significant variation in flow velocities during respiration (IN: Start of inspiration). Later the same day 800 ml of blood was evacuated from the pericardial sac.

record, and reopening after atrial contraction may be interpreted as marking the end of the Pc/To interval. Significant overestimation of the pulmonary artery pressure may then occur. The shape of the velocity curve in the pulmonary artery may be of help by indicating the level of pulmonary hypertension [39, 40]. However, the shape is also influenced by other factors [1].

The accuracy of the methods, especially the two first mentioned, provides the clinician a completely noninvasive method to monitor the pulmonary artery pressure. The importance of having several methods at disposition, is that one will act as a control of the other(s). The impact on pediatric cardiology is obvious, but even in adult patients the methods are very useful. The estimation of right sided pressures is part of the complete noninvasive evaluation of patients with valvular and myocardial diseases.

Conclusions

With Doppler cardiography, a powerful and noninvasive tool for the evaluation of hemodynamic changes in various heart diseases has become available. However, to be able to rely on the method, the examination technique and technical equipment must be of a high standard.

One great advantage is that the information obtained is complementary to that obtained by echocardiography. In adult cardiology, coronary artery disease remains the only disease where catheterization is definitively superior to noninvasive examination with Doppler and echocardiography.

References

1. Hatle L, Angelsen B: Doppler ultrasound in cardiology (2nd ed.) Philadelphia: Lea & Febiger, 1985.

2. Holen J, Aaslid R, Landmark K, Simonsen S: Determination of pressure gradient in mitral stenosis with a noninvasive ultrasound Doppler technique. Act Med Scan 199: 455–60, 1976.
3. Hatle L, Brubakk A, Tromsdal A, Angelsen B: Noninvasive assessment of pressure drop in mitral stenosis by Doppler ultrasound. Br Heart J 40: 131–40, 1978.
4. Hegrenaes L, Hatle L: Aortic stenosis in adults. Non-invasive estimation of pressure differences by continuous wave Doppler echocardiography. Br Heart J 54: 396–404, 1985.
5. Currie PJ, Seward JB, Reeder GS, Vlietstra RE, Bresnahan DR, Bresnahan JF, Smith HC, Hagler DJ, Tajik AJ: Continuous-wave Doppler echocardiographic assessment of severity of calcific aortic stenosis: a simultaneous Doppler-catheter correlative study in 100 adult patients. Circulation 71: 1162–1169, 1985.
6. Teirstein PS, Yock PG, Popp RL: The accuracy of Doppler ultrasound measurement of pressure gradients across irregular, dual, and tunnellike obstructions to blood flow. Circulation 72: 577–584, 1985.
7. Smith MD, Dawson PL, Elion JL, Booth DC, Handshoe R, Kwan OL, Earle GF, DeMaria AN: Correlation of continuous wave Doppler Velocities with cardiac catheterization gradients: An experimental modal of aortic stenosis. J Am Coll Cardiol 6: 1306–1314, 1985.
8. Oliveira Lima C, Sahn DJ, Valdes-Cruz LM, Goldberg SJ, Vargas Barron J, Allen HD, Grenadier E: Noninvasive prediction of transvalvular pressure gradient in patients with pulmonary stenosis by quantitative two-dimensional echo Doppler studies. Circulation 67: 866–871, 1983.
9. Hatle L, Angelsen B, Tromsdal A: Noninvasive assessment of atrioventricular pressure half-time by Doppler ultrasound. Circulation 60: 1096–1104, 1979.
10. Kosturakis D, Allen HD, Goldberg SJ, Sahn DJ, Valdes-Cruz LM: Noninvasive quantification of stenotic semilunar valve areas by Doppler echocardiography. J Am Coll Cardiol 3: 1256–1262, 1984.
11. Fujii K, Kitabatake A, Asao M, Tanouchi J, Ishihara K, Morita T, Masuyama T, Ito H, Hori M, Inoue M, Abe H: Noninvasive evaluation of valvular stenosis by a quantitive Doppler technique. Abstract. J Cardiov Ultrasonography 3: 201, 1984.
12. Skjaerpe T, Hegrenaes L, Hatle L: Noninvasive estimation of valve area in patients with aortic stenosis by Doppler ultrasound and two-dimensional echocardiography. Circulation 72: 810–818, 1985.
13. Rodrigo FA: Estimation of valve area and 'valvular resistance'. A critical study of the physical basis of the methods employed. Am Heart J 45: 1–12, 1953.
14. Hatle L: Noninvasive assessment and differentiation of left ventricular outflow obstruction by Doppler ultrasound. Circulation 64: 381–387, 1981.
15. Wautrecht JC, Vandenbossche JL, Englert M: Sensitivity and specificity of pulsed Doppler echocardiography in detection of aortic and mitral regurgitation. Eur Heart J 5: 404–411, 1984.
16. Miyatake K, Okamoto M, Kinoshita N, Matushisa M, Nagata S, Beppu S, Park Y, Sakakibara H, Nimura Y: Pulmonary regurgitation studied with the ultrasonic pulsed Doppler technique. Circulation 65: 970–976, 1982.
17. Miyatake K, Okamoto M, Kinoshita N, Ohta M, Kozuka T, Sakakibara H, Nimura Y: Evaluation of tricuspid regurgitation by pulsed Doppler and two-dimensional echoardiography. Circulation 66: 777–83, 1982.
18. Skjaerpe T, Hatle L: Diagnosis and assessment of tricuspid regurgitation with Doppler ultrasound pp. 299–304. In : Rijsterborgh H (ed.) Echocardiology. The Hague: Martinus Nijhoff Publishers, 1981.
19. Skjaerpe T, Hatle L: Diagnosis of tricuspid regurgitation. Sensitivity of Doppler ultrasound compared with contrast echocardiography. Eur Heart J 6: 429–436, 1985.
20. Samstad S, Hegrenaes H, Haugland T, Nordby A, Skjaerpe T: Evaluation of aortic and mitral regurgitation with Doppler ultrasound and cineangiography – A comparative study of two semiquantitative techniques. J Cardiov Ultrasonography IV: Abstract, 1985.

21. Croft CH, Lipscomb K, Mathis K, Firth BG, Nicod P, Tilton G, Winniford MD, Hillis LD: Limitations of qualitative angiographic grading in aortic or mitral regurgitation. Am J Cardiol 53: 1593–1598, 1984.
22. Wranne B, Ask P, Loyd D: Factors influencing fluid velocity in valve regurgitations. Ultrasonoor bulletin special issue: 82 (Abstract), 1985.
23. Hatle L, Samstad S, Hegrenaes L, Skjaerpe T: Pressure half-time in aortic regurgitation from Doppler – A measure of the severity? Abstract. J Cardiov Ultrasonography IV, 1985.
24. Diebold B, Touati R, Blanchard D, Colonna G, Guermonprez JL, Peronneau P, Forman J, Maurice P: Quantitative assessment of tricuspid regurgitation using pulsed Doppler echocardiography. Br Heart J 50: 443–449, 1983.
25. Saksi K, Nakamura K, Satomi G, Kondo M, Hirosawa K: Evaluation of tricuspid regurgitation by blood flow pattern in the hepatic vein using pulsed Doppler technique. Am Heart J 108: 516–523, 1984.
26. Diebold B, Peronneau P, Blanchard D, Colonna G, Guermonprez JL, Forman J, Sellier P, Maurice P: Noninvasive quantification of aortic regurgitation by Doppler echocardiography. Br Heart J 49: 167–173, 1983.
27. Zhang Y, Ihlen H, Myhre E, Levorstad K, Nitter-Hauge S: Measurement of mitral regurgitation by Doppler echocardiography. Br Heart J 54: 384–391, 1985.
28. Kitabatake A, Ito H, Inoue M, Tanouchi J, Ishihara K, Morita T, Fujii K, Yoshida Y, Masuyama T, Yoshima H, Hori M, Kamada T: A new approach to noninvasive evaluation of aortic regurgitant fraction by two-dimensional Doppler echocardiography. Circulation 72: 523–529, 1985.
29. Lewis JF, Kuo LC, Nelson JG, Limacher MC, Quinones MA: Pulsed Doppler echocardiographic determination of stroke volume and cardiac output: Clinical validation of two new methods using the apical window. Circulation 70: 425, 1984.
30. Ihlen H, Amlie JP, Dale J, Forfang K, Nitter-Hauge S, Otterstad JE, Simonsen S, Myhre E: Determination of cardiac output by Doppler echocardiography. Br Heart J 51: 54–60, 1984.
31. Goldberg SJ, Sahn DJ, Allen HD, Valdes-Cruz LM, Hoenecke H, Carnahan Y: Evaluation of pulmonary and systemic blood flow by 2-dimensional Doppler echocardiography using fast Fourier transform spectral analysis. Am J Cardiol 50: 1394–1400, 1982.
32. Sanders SP, Yeager S, Williams RG: Measurements of systemic and pulmonary blood flow and QP/QS ratio using Doppler and two-dimensional echocardiography. Am J Cardiol 51: 952–956, 1983.
33. Loeppky JA, Hoekenga DE, Greene ER, Luft UC: Comparison of noninvasive pulsed Doppler and Fick measurements of stroke volume in cardiac patients. Am Heart J 107: 33–37, 1984.
34. Huntsman LL, Stewart DK, Barnes SR, Franklin SB, Colocousis JS, Hessel EA: Noninvasive Doppler determination of cardiac output in man. Clinical validation. Circulation 67: 593–602, 1983.
35. Skjaerpe T: Influence of the geometry of the ascending aorta upon the velocity profile. In: Spencer MP (ed.) Cardiac Doppler diagnosis, Volume II. Boston: Martinus Nijhoff Publishers, 1986.
36. Gisvold SE, Brubakk AO: Measurements of instantaneous blood-flow velocity in the human aorta using pulsed ultrasound. Cardiovasc Res 16: 26–33, 1982.
37. Light LH, Sequiera RF, Cross G, Bilton A, Hanson GC: Flow oriented circulatory patients assessment and management using transcutaneous aortovelography, a noninvasive Doppler technique. J Nucl Med Allied Sci 23: 137–144, 1979.
38. Hatle L, Angelsen BAJ, Tromsdal A: Noninvasive estimation of pulmonary artery systolic pressure with Doppler ultrasound. Br Heart J 45: 157–165, 1981.
39. Redel D, Victor S: Pulsed Doppler echocardiography – a noninvasive method for assessment of pulmonary hypertension. World Congress of Pediatric Cardiology, 1980: 323 (Abstract).
40. Kitabatake A, Inoue M, Asao M, Masuyama T, Tanouchi J, Morita T, Mishima M, Uematsu M,

Shimazu T, Hori M, Abe H: Noninvasive evaluation of pulmonary hypertension by a pulsed Doppler technique. Circulation 68: 302–309, 1983.

41. Skjaerpe T, Hatle L: Noninvasive estimation of pulmonary artery pressure by Doppler ultrasound in tricuspid regurgitation. In: Spencer MP (ed.) Cardiac Doppler diagnosis, pp. 247–54. Boston: Martinus Nijhoff Publishers, 1983.

42. Yock PG, Popp RL: Noninvasive estimation of right ventricular systolic pressure by Doppler ultrasound in patients with tricuspid regurgitation. Circulation 70: 657–62, 1984.

43. Currie PJ, Seward JB, Chan KL, Fyfe DA, Hagler DJ, Mair DD, Reeder GS, Nishimura RA, Tajik AJ: Continuous wave Doppler determination of right ventricular pressure: A simultaneous Doppler-catheterization study in 127 patients. J Am Coll Cardiol 6: 750–756, 1985.

44. Berger M, Haimowitz A, Van Tosh A, Berdoff RL, Goldberg E: Quantitative assessment of pulmonary hypertension in patients with tricuspid regurgitation using continuous wave Doppler ultrasound. J Am Coll Cardiol 6: 359–365, 1985.

Limitations of Doppler measurement of volume flow in adults with aortic stenosis

Catherine M. Otto*, Alan S. Pearlman, Keith A. Comess*, A. Kim Saal, Carolyn L. Janko and Robyn R. Reamer

Abstract

Transvalvular gradients, which can be measured by Doppler in patients with aortic stenosis, vary with volume flow. Therefore, we tested three Doppler methods for measuring stroke volume (SV) in adults with aortic stenosis undergoing catheterization. Doppler velocities and 2D echo images were recorded immediately post-cath, simultaneous with thermodilution (TD) cardiac output. Doppler stroke volume was calculated from vessel diameter and the integral of the flow velocity curve. Using pulmonary artery flow and diameter, agreement between Doppler and TD was good (r = 0.83, DOP = 1.1 TD + 5.2 ml), but diameter could be recorded in only 15/48 (31%) patients. Mitral annular diameter and left ventricular inflow could be recorded in 41/48 (85%), but agreement with TD stroke volume was only fair (r = 0.63, DOP = 1.5 TD − 8.1 ml). Moreover, the mitral annulus method was rendered inappropriate by the high prevalence of mitral regurgitation (83%) in this group. Finally, coexisting aortic insufficiency was present in over 80% of our patients and was more than trivial in 66%. In this situation, a measure of actual transaortic flow is needed since neither pulmonary artery flow nor left ventricular filling represents total transaortic flow. Ascending aortic volume flow cannot be measured because it is non-laminar.

To circumvent these difficulties, we measured left ventricular outflow tract (LVOT) diameter and flow just below the stenotic aortic valve. These measures were feasible in 47/49 (96%) patients. In the 38 patients with LV angiograms, the Doppler LVOT stroke volume was compared to angio stroke volume (r = 0.69, DOP = 0.59 Angio + 36.1 ml). In the last 12 patients, the correlation of the LVOT stroke volume with angio stroke volume was improved (r = 0.85), which may represent a learning effect.

We conclude that in adults with aortic stenosis

* Grant support: Dr Otto and Dr Comess were research fellows of the American Heart Association, Washington Affiliate.

1. the pulmonary artery method measures TD-SV accurately, but it cannot be used in the majority of patients;
2. the mitral annulus method does not provide an accurate measure of volume flow; and
3. although the agreement between the LVOT method and angio-SV has not been ideal, this method does measure transaortic flow and can be recorded in nearly all patients, and so merits further evaluation.

Introduction

Transvalvular gradients, which can be measured by Doppler in patients with aortic stenosis [1–5], vary with volume flow. Thus noninvasive determination of the severity of stenosis (best expressed as aortic valve area) requires measurement of both transaortic pressure gradient and transaortic volume flow.

Volume flow can be measured by Doppler and two-dimensional echocardiography as the cross-sectional area of flow times the mean flow velocity during the period of flow, assuming that flow is laminar and has a flat velocity profile across the vessel lumen. This method has been used to measure volume flow in the ascending aorta, left ventricular outflow tract, pulmonary artery, and across the mitral and tricuspid valves in patients without significant valvular disease [7–11]. Using Doppler methods, volume flow can be measured only at those intracardiac sites where flow remains laminar [12]. In aortic stenosis, volume flow cannot be measured in the ascending aorta because of turbulence distal to the stenotic valve. Therefore, we tested Doppler measurement of volume flow in adults with aortic stenosis at three other intracardiac sites: 1. pulmonary artery, 2. mitral annulus, and 3. left ventricular outflow tract proximal to the stenotic valve. Each Doppler method was compared to forward stroke volume measured simultaneously by thermodilution and to total stroke volume measured by angiography.

Methods

Patient population

Doppler and 2D echo studies were performed immediately post-catheterization in 66 adults with suspected aortic stenosis. A thermodilution catheter was left in position in the pulmonary artery for simultaneous measurement of cardiac output. Patients ranged in age from 33 to 84 years (mean age 66 years), with 48 males and 18 females. All three methods for calculation of volume flow were performed in 31 patients. An additional 17 had the pulmonary artery and mitral annulus measures, for a total of 40 studies using these two methods. In an additional 18, only LVOT meaures were performed, for a total of 49 studies with this method. Informed consent was obtained in all patients.

Cardiac catheterization

Cardiac catheterization was performed for clinical indications. The left ventricular (LV) to aortic pressure gradient was measured with fluid-filled catheters connected to Stratham P23d B transducers. Forward cardiac output was measured in triplicate by thermodilution using 10 cc boluses of iced saline and an Edwards Laboratories cardiac output computer with strip chart recorder. Total stroke volume was calculated from single-plane left ventricular angiography in a 30° RAO position [13]. Aortic valve area was calculated using the Gorlin formula [14].

Echo-Doppler

At ATL 600 (Advanced Technologies Laboratories, Bothell, WA) instrument was used for two-dimensional (2D) and pulsed Doppler echocardiography. Two-dimensional images for measurement of diameter at each intracardiac site were recorded on videotape. The Doppler flow curve was recorded on videotape and on paper at 50 mm/s. A 9 mm sample volume length was used to provide a degree of spatial averaging. The Doppler signal was optimized by careful transducer positioning and angulation, in order to obtain a tonal audible signal with a smooth signal envelope on spectral analysis and flow with the highest peak. This flow was assumed to have been obtained at a near-parallel intercept angle, so a value of 1 was used for cos θ in the Doppler equation:

$$v = \frac{c(f_2 - f_1)}{2f_1 \cos \theta}$$

where v = blood flow velocity (m/s), c = speed of sound in blood (1540 m/s), f_1 = carrier frequency (KHz), $(f_2 - f_1)$ = Doppler shift (KHz) and θ = angle between the ultrasound beam and direction of blood flow.

Pulmonary artery diameter was measured from parasternal 2D images oriented in the long axis of the pulmonary artery. The pulmonary artery systolic velocity curve was recorded with the sample volume positioned in the center of the vessel distal to the valve (Fig. 1).

The mitral annulus diameter was recorded from both apical four-chamber and two-chamber views. The diastolic transmitral flow velocity curve was recorded with the sample volume positioned in the center of the annulus. The sample volume was then positioned to show the highest velocity LV filling curve, which

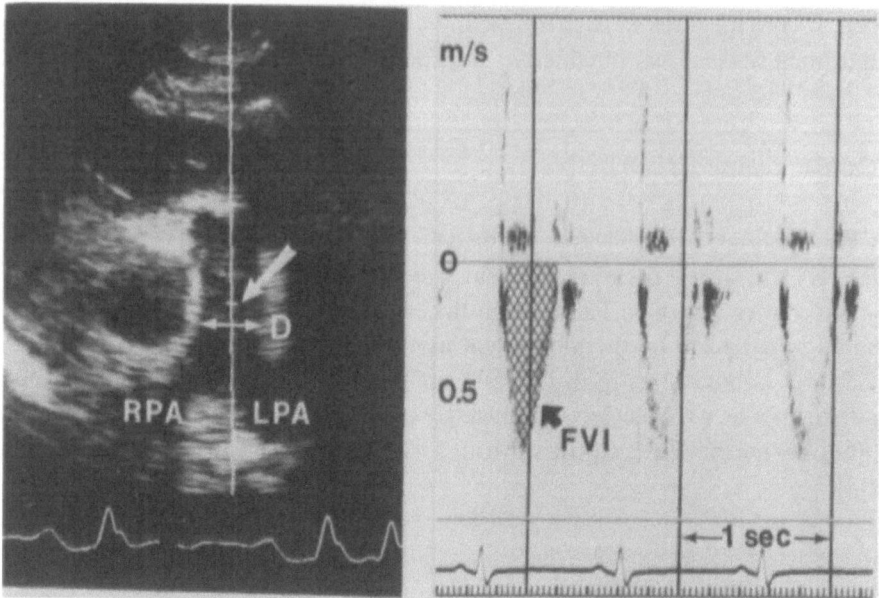

Figure 1. Pulmonary artery method: On the left, diameter (D) was measured from a parasternal long-axis view of the pulmonary artery, and cross-sectional area calculated as $\pi \left(\frac{D}{2}\right)^2$. The pulsed Doppler sample volume was positioned in the main pulmonary artery as shown (arrow). On the right, the systolic velocity curve was integrated with respect to time as indicated by the cross-hatched area on the spectral analysis. Stroke volume (SV) was calculated as the cross-sectional area time the flow velocity integral. RPA = right pulmonary artery, LPA = left pulmonary artery.

was usually closer to the mitral leaflet tips (Fig. 2).

Left ventricular outflow tract (LVOT) diameter was measured from parasternal long-axis images. LVOT flow was recorded from an apical long-axis or five-chamber view with the sample volume positioned just proximal to the stenotic valve (Fig. 3).

The inner-edge to inner-edge diameter (D) at each intracardiac site was averaged from five to ten video images using a calibrated video overlay system. The cross-sectional area (CSA) of flow was calculated as $\pi \left(\frac{D}{2}\right)^2$, assuming the area of flow to be circular. The flow velocity integral (FVI) was averaged from three to five beats (eight to ten beats if atrial fibrillation was present) using a Franklin Insight 2000 (Franklin, Inc., Woodinville, WA) to integrate the Doppler velocity curve over the period of flow.

For each intracardiac site, stroke volume (SV) was calculated as:

$$SV \ (cm^3) = CSA \ (cm^2) \times FVI \ (cm)$$

A thermodilution cardiac output was obtained in triplicate twice during the

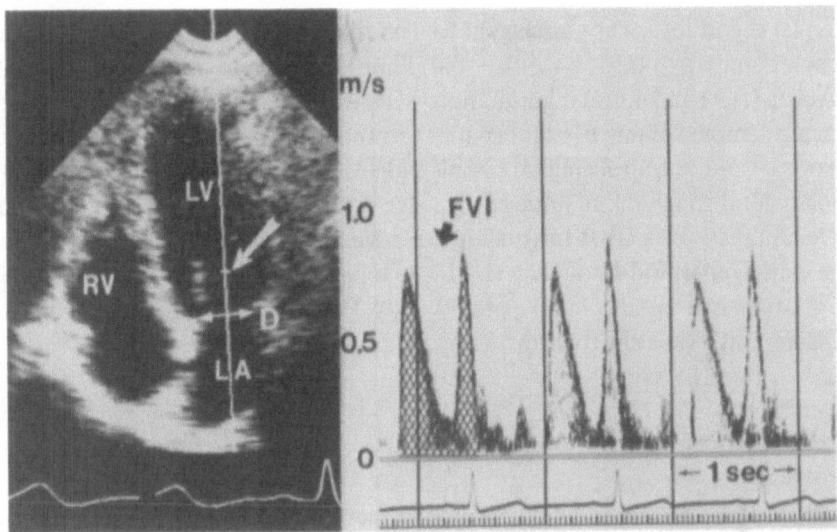

Figure 2. Mitral annulus method: On the left, mitral annulus diameter was measured from an apical four-chamber view as shown. The sample volume (arrow) was positioned to record the highest velocity left ventricular filling curve. On the right, the diastolic flow velocity curve was integrated (FVI) with respect to time as shown by the cross-hatched area.

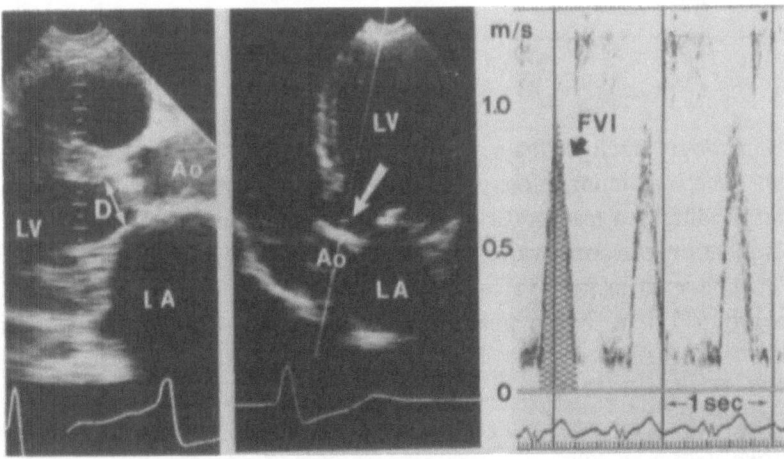

Figure 3. Left ventricular outflow tract method: Left: LVOT internal diameter was measured in mid-systole just below the stenotic aortic valve as shown. Center: LVOT flow was recorded from the apex with the sample volume (arrow) positioned just proximal to the aortic valve. Right: The Doppler spectral analysis is shown with the display inverted and the baseline at the bottom. The area under the systolic flow curve was measured as shown by the cross-hatched area.

Doppler recordings. The two sets showed no changes in cardiac output during the Doppler study (r = 0.95, y = 1.0x − 0.07 l/min). Heart rate also was unchanged.

Aortic (AR) and mitral regurgitation (MR) were mapped with pulsed Doppler (1.5 mm sample volume used for spatial accuracy) and graded as mild, moderate or severe [15–17]. Mitral annular calcification was noted on 2D images. The high-velocity jet through the stenotic aortic valve was recorded using both continuous wave Doppler (Irex III-B instrument; Irex Medical Systems, Ramsey, NJ) and high pulse repetition frequency (HPRF) Doppler (ATL-600 instrument) in 50 (76%) patients. In 16 (24%) patients only HPRF Doppler was available to measure aortic jet velocity [18].

Data analysis

Stroke volume measured by each Doppler method was compared to 1. forward stroke volume, measured simultaneously by thermodilution and 2. total stroke volume, determined nonsimultaneously by angiography. Linear regression with calculation of Pearson's correlation coefficient was used for statistical analysis. The same observer made all echo-Doppler measurements blinded to the angiographic and thermodilution results. Intra- and interobserver variability for measurement of the Doppler flow velocity integral and the 2D diameter was less than 6%, using the mean coefficient of variation.

Results

Severity of aortic stenosis

The maximum velocity in the aortic jet ranged from 1.6 to 5.4 m/s with a mean of 3.4 m/s. The maximum velocity was greater than 3.6 m/s in 38 (58%) patients (corresponding to a transaortic gradient $\geqslant$ 50 mmHg, calculated as $4(V_{max})^2$. At catheterization, the aortic valve area ranged from 0.3 to 3.7 (mean 0.9) cm^2, with 47 (71%) patients having a valve area $\leqslant$ 1.0 cm^2. Of note, 9 patients with an aortic valve area $\leqslant$ 1.0 cm^2 had a pressure gradient < 50 mmHg because transaortic volume flow was low.

Pulmonary artery method

Stroke volume by the pulmonary artery Doppler method compared well to simultaneous forward stroke volume by thermodilution (r = 0.83, DOP = 1.1 TD + 5.2 ml, SEE = 15.0 ml; Fig. 4). However, this method could be performed in only 15/48 (31%) due to inability to image the pulmonary artery diameter in the

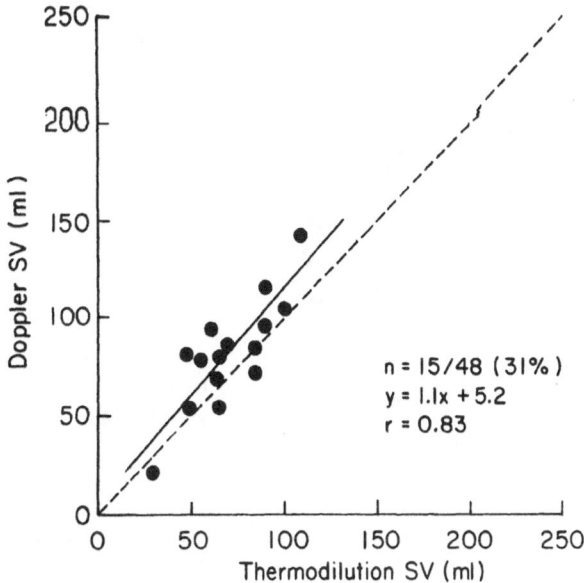

Figure 4. Pulmonary artery method: The Doppler stroke volume (y-axis) is compared by linear regression to simultaneous thermodilution stroke volume (x-axis). The regression line (solid) and the line of identity (dashed) are shown.

remaining patients. Correlation with total stroke volume by angiography was poor ($r = 0.12$).

Mitral annulus method

The mitral annulus method was feasible in 41/48 (85%) since the apical window provided ultrasound access for both 2D imaging of mitral annulus diameter and Doppler recording of transmitral flow in most patients. However, the correlation of Doppler transmitral stroke volume with simultaneous forward stroke volume by thermodilution was only fair ($r = 0.63$, DOP = 1.5 TD − 8.1 ml, SEE = 36.0 ml; Fig. 5). The correlation was not improved by assuming an elliptical mitral annulus and using diameters measured in two orthogonal planes ($r = 0.64$), or by using the Doppler flow velocity curve recorded with the sample volume positioned at the annulus ($r = 0.55$) instead of the highest velocity transmitral flow (which usually was found nearer the leaflet tips).

The transmitral flow velocity curve was recorded in all patients, but mitral annulus diameter could not be measured properly in seven – three with mild mitral stenosis, two with suboptimal images due to poor ultrasound tissue penetration, and two with severe mitral annular calcification. In fact, mitral annular-calcification was common in this population (23/48, 48%), which made accurate

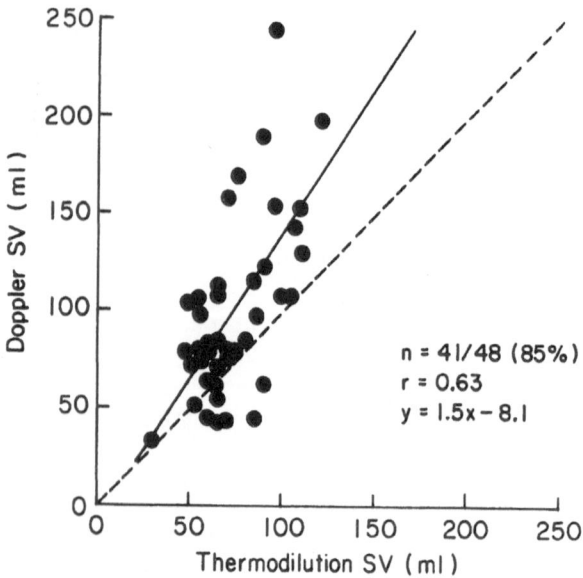

Figure 5. Mitral annulus method: The Doppler stroke volume (y-axis) using a circular mitral annulus and the highest velocity LV-filling curve is compared by linear regression to simultaneous thermodilution stroke volume (x-axis).

measurement of mitral annulus diameter difficult in many cases. In addition, mitral regurgitation was present in 41/48 (85%) patients and was mild in 27 (56% of total), moderate in 14 (29% of total) and severe in none. Transmitral stroke volume did not correlate well ($r = 0.38$) with total stroke volume by angiography in our population.

Coexisting aortic regurgitation

Aortic regurgitation was detected by Doppler in 54/66 (82%) of these patients with suspected aortic stenosis. The severity of AR was mild in 11, moderate in 31 and severe in 12. Thus, of those with AR, 43/66 (66%) had more than trivial regurgitation.

Left ventricular outflow tract (LVOT) method

Measurement of LVOT diameter was possible in all patients, and ranged from 1.7 to 3.5 (mean 2.4) cm. An LVOT flow velocity curve was recorded in 47/49 (96%) patients. The two failures were due to turbulent LVOT flow; one of these patients also had a high membranous ventricular septal defect. LVOT flow was recorded from the apex at a depth of 11 cm in 17, 13 cm in 25 and 15 cm in 5 patients. The maximum velocity in the LVOT ranged from 0.5 to 1.8 m/s (mean 0.9 m/s). HPRF Doppler was needed in three patients to record LVOT flow without aliasing.

The LVOT stroke volume by Doppler correlated poorly with the forward stroke volume by thermodilution (r = 0.34). An angiographic total stroke volume was available in 38/49 (78%) of the patients. The correlation between the Doppler LVOT method and the non-simultaneous angiographic stroke volume is shown in Figure 6 (n = 38, r = 0.69, Dop = 0.59 Angio + 36.1 ml, SEE = 25.0 ml). The correlation in the last 12 patients studied was higher (r = 0.85) than in the total group.

Overlap group

Results in the subgroup of 31 patients in whom all three methods were attempted are similar to those reported above. The pulmonary artery method was possible in 10/31 (32%), the mitral annulus method in 26/31 (84%) and the LVOT method in 30/31 (97%). Correlations with thermodilution stroke volume for pulmonary artery (r = 0.77) and mitral annulus (r = 0.55), and angiographic stroke volume for LVOT (r = 0.64) were similar in this subgroup to results in the total group.

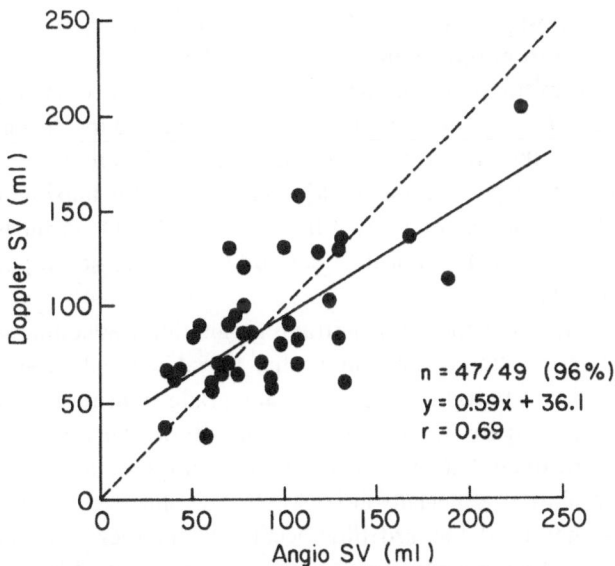

Figure 6. Left ventricular outflow tract method: The Doppler transaortic stroke volume (y-axis) is compared by linear regression to the angiographic stroke volume (x-axis). Adequate 2D and Doppler echo data were recorded in 47/49 patients, although angiograms were available for comparison in only 38.

Discussion

Since pressure gradient depends on volume flow, a noninvasive method to measure transaortic volume flow is needed for accurate assessment of the severity of aortic stenosis. In this study, we evaluated three Doppler-echo methods for measurement of volume flow in adults with aortic stenosis.

Measures of stroke volume in the pulmonary artery compare well to simultaneous forward stroke volume. However this method is feasible in only about one-third of patients due to inability to image the lateral wall of the pulmonary artery in order to measure its diameter. Also, this method correlates poorly with total left ventricular stroke volume.

Measurement of transmitral stroke volume is technically possible in most patients, but correlation with forward or total stroke volume is poor. The Doppler method relies on several assumptions. Difficulty measuring mitral annulus diameter precisely – due to the limited lateral resolution of the ultrasound beam as well as the presence of mitral annular calcification in many patients – may account for part of the discrepancy between Doppler and thermodilution stroke volumes. The assumption that the mitral annulus is circular in cross-section may be an oversimplification, but calculation of an elliptical annulus area did not improve the results. Other studies suggest that mitral annulus cross-sectional area changes during diastole, which may also lead to errors in calculation of volume flow [19]. It may also be an oversimplification to assume that, in the absence of mitral stenosis, the mitral annulus is the limiting orifice to left ventricular filling. We noted that, in most patients, the velocity of LV filling increased as the sample volume was moved from the annulus towards the leaflet tips. Again, however, calculation of transmitral stroke volume using diameter and flow measured at the same anatomic site (at the annulus) did not improve the results. Attempts to use the mitral orifice method described by Fischer et al. [20] were unsuccessful in a small subgroup of these patients due to difficulty imaging the maximum diastolic mitral valve orifice on parasternal views. In addition, although the measurements were done carefully and in triplicate, thermodilution cardiac outputs are not always accurate [21].

Of more concern is that coexisting mitral regurgitation was common (85%) in these adults with aortic stenosis, and more than trivial in about one-third. In the presence of significant mitral regurgitation, antegrade transmitral volume flow would not be expected to equal forward volume flow. This may explain the tendency to 'overestimate' stroke volume by the mitral annulus method compared to thermodilution, especially at larger stroke volumes.

Even if they measured forward flow accurately, neither transpulmonic of transmitral volume flow is equivalent to trans-aortic volume flow when aortic regurgitation is present. In this situation (AR was present in 82% and more than mild in 2/3 of our population) transaortic volume flow is better measured as total stroke volume (as is calculated by angiography) rather than forward stroke volume (as is determined by indicator-dilution, or Fick methods).

Transaortic volume flow cannot be measured in the ascending aorta using echo/ Doppler methods because flow is disturbed distal to the stenotic aortic valve. However, we hypothesized that since flow proximal to a stenosis is thought to be laminar and normal in velocity, transaortic stroke volume could be measured in the left ventricular outflow tract proximal to the valve. This method was technically feasible in nearly all patients, and results compared to angiographic stroke volume were encouraging. In addition, there may be a learning curve effect for recording LVOT diameter and flow optimally, since the results in the last 12 patients were better than in the group as a whole. We believe that the lack of a better correlation between the Doppler-echo method and angiography may be due to limitations in both techniques.

The Doppler-echo method makes several assumptions about LVOT geometry and flow. The LVOT is assumed to be circular just below the stenotic valve and to remain constant in area during systole. Short-axis 2D images support this approximation. Since LVOT diameter is measured with the ultrasound beam perpendicular to its wall, accurate and repeatable diameter measurement is more likely than with pulmonary artery or mitral annulus. Flow is assumed to fill the anatomic LVOT and to be laminar with a flat velocity profile.

An adequate angiogram for calculation of transaortic stroke volume was not obtained in all patients (78% technically adequate angiograms versus 96% technically adequate echo-Doppler studies). Moreover, some of the LV angiograms were via a left atrial injection so mitral regurgitation could not be evaluated. In order to avoid bias based on the Doppler findings, we assumed that the total LV stroke volume was equal to transaortic flow; no correction was made for the fraction of the total stroke volume due to mitral regurgitation. Since mitral regurgitation was common by Doppler, this may have led to overestimation of transaortic flow by angiography in some individuals. Even under ideal circumstances the accuracy of angiographic stroke volumes is $\pm 7\%$ [13].

Finally the Doppler and angiographic recordings were not simultaneous. Rigorous validation of the LVOT method will require simultaneous, accurate, direct measures of transaortic volume flow and the ability to vary volume flow for a given aortic valve area.

We conclude that in adults with aortic stenosis, echo-Doppler measurement of volume flow is not simple. The pulmonary artery method measures forward stroke volume accurately but is seldom feasible. The mitral annulus method correlates less well with forward stroke volume. Neither of these two methods measures transaortic flow, and since coexisting aortic insufficiency is common in adults with aortic stenosis, measures of forward stroke volume are inadequate. Although the agreement between the LVOT method and angiography is only fair, this method does measure transaortic flow, and it can be applied to nearly all patients. Previous work has shown that measurement of LVOT flow in combination with measurement of the aortic jet provides a better index of the severity of aortic stenosis than pressure gradient alone [20]. Further evaluation of the LVOT method is merited, as it may allow fully noninvasive determination of aortic valve area in adults with AS.

References

1. Hatle L, Angelsen BA, Tromsdal A: Non-invasive assessment of aortic stenosis by Doppler ultrasound. Br Heart J 43: 284–292, 1980.
2. Hatle L: Noninvasive assessment and differentiation of left ventricular outflow obstruction with Doppler ultrasound. Circulation 64: 381–387, 1981.
3. Lima CO, Sahn DJ, Valdes-Cruz LM, Allen HD, Goldberg SJ, Grenadier E, Barron JV: Prediction of the severity of left ventricular outflow tract obstruction by quantitative two-dimensional echocardiographic studies. Circulation 68: 348–354, 1983.
4. Stamm RB, Martin RP. Quantification of pressure gradients across stenotic valves by Doppler ultrasound. J Am Coll Cardiol 2: 707–718, 1983.
5. Berger M, Berdoff RL, Gallerstein PE, Goldberg E: Evaluation of aortic stenosis by continuous wave Doppler ultrasound. J Am Coll Cardiol 3: 150–156, 1984.
6. Stevenson JG, Kawabori I: Noninvasive determination of pressure gradients in children: Two methods employing pulsed Doppler echocardiography. J Am Coll Cardiol 3: 179–192, 1984.
7. Goldberg SJ, Sahn DJ, Allen HD, Valdes-Cruz LM, Hoenecke J, Carnahan Y: Evaluation of pulmonary and systemic blood flow by two dimensional Doppler echocardiography using fast Fourier transform spectral analysis. Am J Cardiol 50: 1394–1400, 1982.
8. Huntsman LL, Stewart DK, Barnes SR, Franklin SB, Colocousis JS, Hessel EA: Non-invasive Doppler determination of cardiac output in man: Clinical validation. Circulation 67: 593–601, 1983.
9. Sanders SP, Yeager S, Williams RG: Measurement of systemic and pulmonary blood flow and QP/QS ratio using Doppler and two-dimensional echocardiography. Am J Cardiol 51: 952–956, 1983.
10. Lewis LF, Kuo LC, Nelson JG, Limacher MC, Quinones MA: Pulsed Doppler echocardiographic determination of stroke volume and cardiac output: Clinical validation of two new methods using the apical window. Circulation 70: 425–431, 1984.
11. Chandraratna PA, Nanna M, McKay C, Nimalasuriya A, Swinney R, Elkayam U, Rahimtoola SH: Determination of cardiac output by transcutaneous continuous-wave ultrasonic Doppler computer. Am J Cardiol 53: 234–237, 1984.
12. Kosturakis D, Allen HD, Goldberg SJ, Sahn DJ, Valdes-Cruz LM: Non-invasive quantification of stenotic semilunar valve areas by Doppler echocardiography. J Am Coll Cardiol 3: 1256–1262, 1984.
13. Sandler H, Dodge HT: The use of single plane angiocardiograms for the calculation of left ventricular volume in man. Am Heart J 75: 325–334, 1968.
14. Gorlin R, Gorlin SG: Hydraulic formula for calculation of the area of the stenotic mitral valve, other cardiac valves, and central circulatory shunts. I. Am Heart J 41: 1–29, 1951.
15. Abbasi AS, Allen M, DeCristofaro D, Ungar I: Detection and estimation of the degree of mitral regurgitation by range-gated pulsed Doppler echocardiography. Circulation 61: 143–147, 1980.
16. Quinones MA, Young JB, Waggoner AD, Ostojic MC, Ribeiro LGT, Miller RR: Assessment of pulsed Doppler echocardiography in detection and quantification of aortic and mitral regurgitation. Br Heart J 44: 612–620, 1980.
17. Ciobanu M, Abbasi AS, Allen M, Hermer A, Spellberg R: Pulsed Doppler echocardiography in the diagnosis and estimation of severity of aortic insufficiency. Am J Cardiol 49: 339–343, 1982.
18. Otto CM, Janko C, Prestley R, Saal AK, Pearlman AS: Measurement of peak blood flow velocity

in adults with valvular aortic stenosis using high pulse repetition frequency duplex pulsed Doppler echocardiography. J Am Coll Cardiol 3: 494 (Abstract), 1984.

19. Ormiston JA, Shah PM, Tei C, Wong M: Size and motion of the mitral valve annulus in man. Circulation 64: 113–120, 1981.

20. Fisher DC, Sahn DJ, Freidman MJ, Larson D, Valdes-Cruz LM, Horowitz S, Goldberg SJ, Allen HD: The mitral valve orifice method for non-invasive two-dimensional echo Doppler determinations of cardiac output. Circulation 67: 872–877, 1983.

21. Schuster AH, Nanda NC: Doppler echocardiographic measurement of cardiac output. Comparison with a non-golden standard. Am J Cardiol 53: 257–259, 1984.

22. Otto CM, Comess KA, Pearlman AS, Reamer RP, Janko CL: Doppler determination of the severity of aortic stenosis in adults. Circulation 70 (II): 115 (Abstract), 1984.

Doppler echocardiographic assessment of normal and malfunctioning mitral valve prostheses

K. Dennig and W. Rudolph

Introduction

The obstruction inherent to prosthetic valves leads to an increase in the velocity of blood flow across the prostheses, which can be detected by Doppler technique and the time profile of which can be characterized by various parameters. Thereby, values of normal functioning prostheses can be evaluated with the aid of which malfunctions may be detected and assessed. This investigation deals with the use of this method as applied to functional assessment of mechanical and biological mitral valve prostheses.

Methods

The studies were carried out in a total of 87 patients after mitral valve replacement – 64 with mechanical Björk-Shiley-monostrut and 23 with Hancock-bioprostheses – in whom normal function at 2–3 weeks post-operatively was documented and 3 patients with prosthetic malfunction, who subsequently underwent cardiac catheterization or reoperation.

Doppler recordings were performed using a 2.0 MHz (PRF 5.74 and 8.62 KHz, maximal velocity limits: ± 1.7 m/s in pulsed and ± 6 m/s in continuous mode) and a 2.4 MHz (PRF 4 and 6 KHz, maximal velocity limits: ± 0.96 m/s in pulsed and ± 7.68 m/s in continuous mode) phased array Doppler echocardiographic system. Velocities recorded were displayed in spectral mode at paper speeds of 50 and 100 mm/s. In all patients the jets through the prostheses were obtained from an apical transducer position.

The Doppler beam was oriented at the audio signal to enable a close alignment with flow direction. No angle corrections were performed at the Doppler system.

Accordingly, as in mitral stenosis, the pressure gradients across the prostheses were calculated by use of the modified Bernoulli equation [1], e.g. the pressure gradient at every point during diastole is derived as 4 times the square of the maximal velocity in the jet through the implant. For this reason, the envelope of the spectral display was interfaced with a computer system, with which the pressure gradient could be printed out as a function of time and the mean diastolic value could be calculated. As an estimate of orifice area the pressure half-time was used, which is the interval of time between the early diastolic peak velocity and the point at which the velocity has been reduced to a value equal to the peak velocity divided by $\sqrt{2}$ [2]. Pressure gradient and half-time were calculated as the mean over 5 diastoles.

Results

The velocity profile of normal functioning mitral valve prostheses was characterized by an early diastolic peak of about 1.5 m/s and a somewhat flatter than normal decrease of the curve from the initial maximum (Figs. 1 and 2). Accordingly, pressure gradients across the mechanical prostheses of 2–4 mmHg were calculated (Fig. 3). Among the various sizes, there was a substantial overlap of data. The pressure gradients for the biological implants with 3–6 mmHg were slightly higher and again, a clear overlap between different sizes were observed (Fig. 4).

The pressure half-times as measured in 64 mechanical prostheses ranged from about 60–90 ms (Fig. 5). There was a relatively small scatter for all sizes and for M 29–33 with mean values of 69 ± 5 (M 29, n = 3), 69 ± 8 (M 31, n = 32) and 72 ± 5 (M 33, n = 27) no significant difference seen (Fig. 6). The pressure half-time for M 27 (n = 2) was with 91 ± 1 ms slightly, but significantly prolonged ($p \leq 0.01$). The pressure half-times in 23 biological prostheses were 118 ± 11 (M 27, n = 2), 87 ± 12 (M 29, n = 3), 80 ± 7 (M 31, n = 10), 73 ± 15 (M 33, n = 4) and 61 ± 2 (M 35, n = 4) ms (Figs. 7 and 8). There was no statistically significant difference between the sizes M 29–33, only the values for M 27 were slightly but significantly longer ($p \leq 0.05$) than those of the other sizes.

In 2 prostheses obstruction was present (Figs. 9 and 10). The substantially increased velocity profiles resulted in pressure gradients of 20 and 6 mmHg, respectively, which were confirmed by hemodynamic measurements. The pressure half-times were prolonged: slightly at 120 ms in the mechanical prosthesis, but substantially at 207 ms in the bioprosthesis.

In one biological prosthesis insufficiency occurred (Fig. 11). The regurgitation into the left atrium was detected by Doppler and the assessment as moderately severe by the mapping method was confirmed by angiography. The calculated pressure value of 9 mmHg correlated well with the invasive value of 8 mmHg. The pressure half-time of 75 ms was within the normal range.

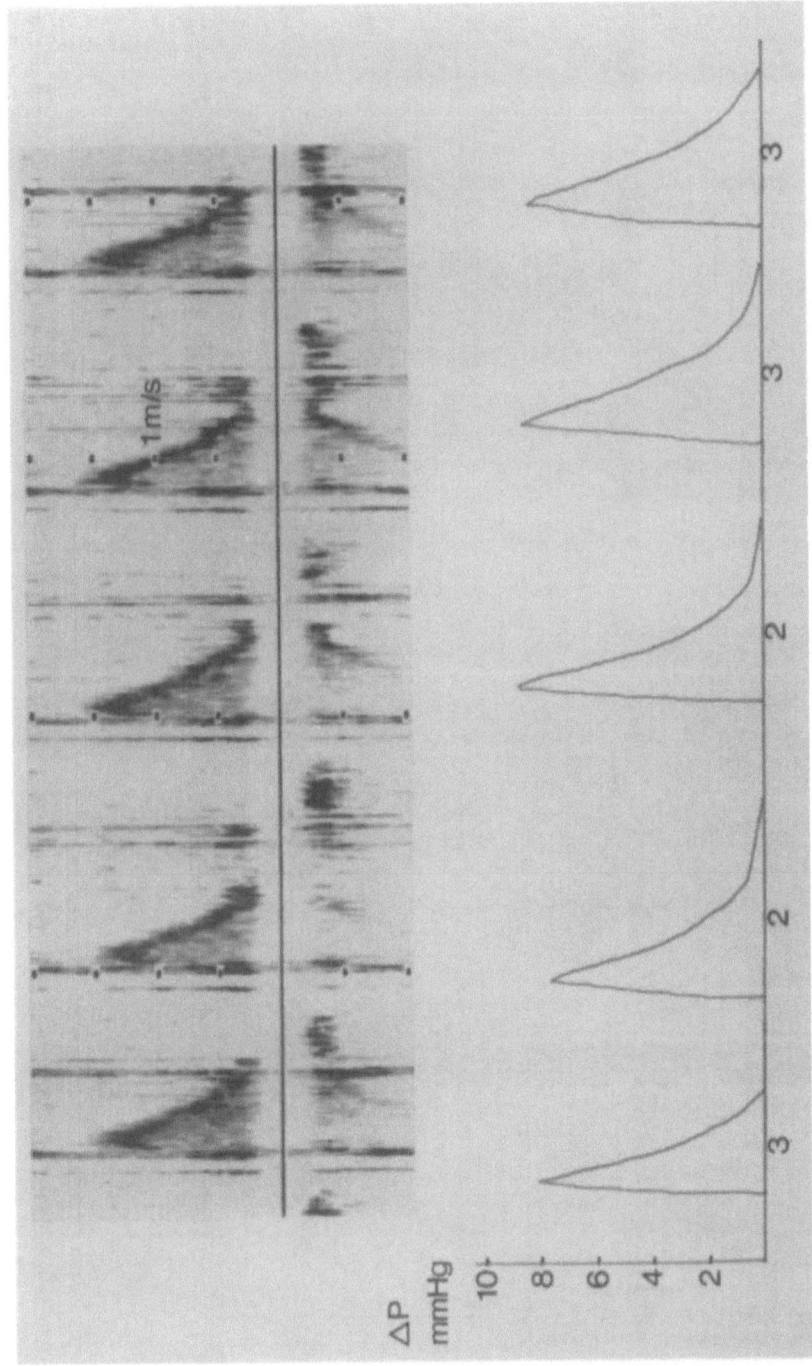

Figure 1. Velocity profile of flow across a mechanical mitral valve prosthesis (Björk-Shiley-monostrut M 31) in the upper panel. Below, the pressure gradients (△P) derived by the Bernoulli equation over each diastole are shown and the mean diastolic gradients are listed.

172

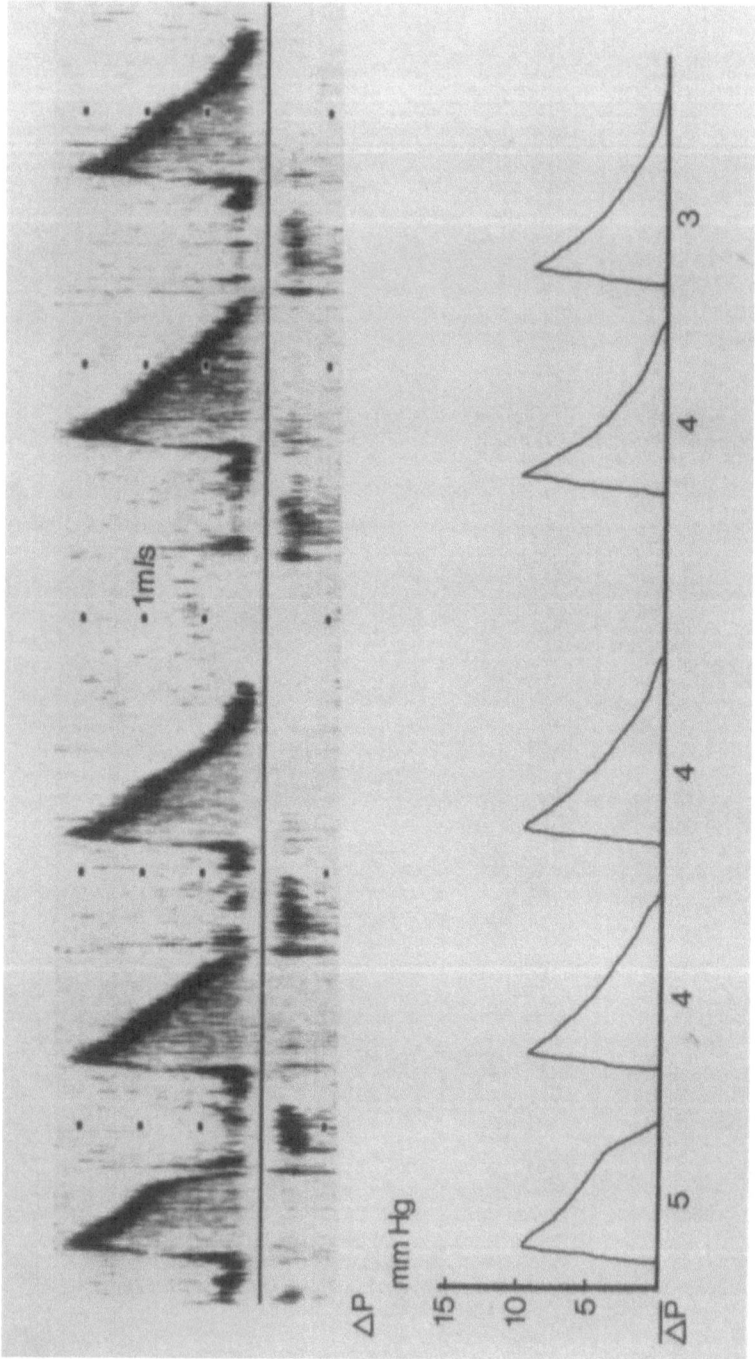

Figure 2. In the upper panel the velocity profile of mitral flow across a biological prosthesis (Hancock M 31) and below the time course of the pressure gradients (△P) as well as the mean diastolic values.

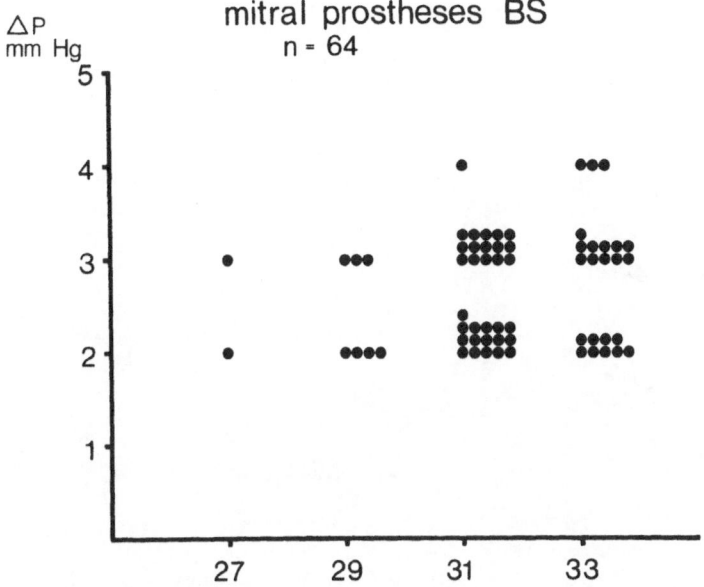

Figure 3. Mean pressure gradients (△P) for various sizes (M 27–33) of 64 Björk-Shiley-monostrut prostheses in mitral position.

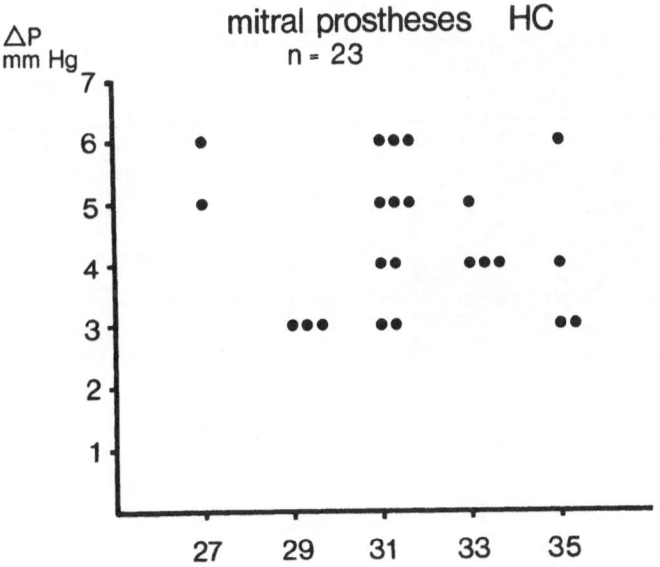

Figure 4. Mean diastolic pressure gradients (△P) of 23 Hancock-bioprostheses in mitral position for various sizes (M 27–33) calculated by the use of the Bernoulli equation.

174

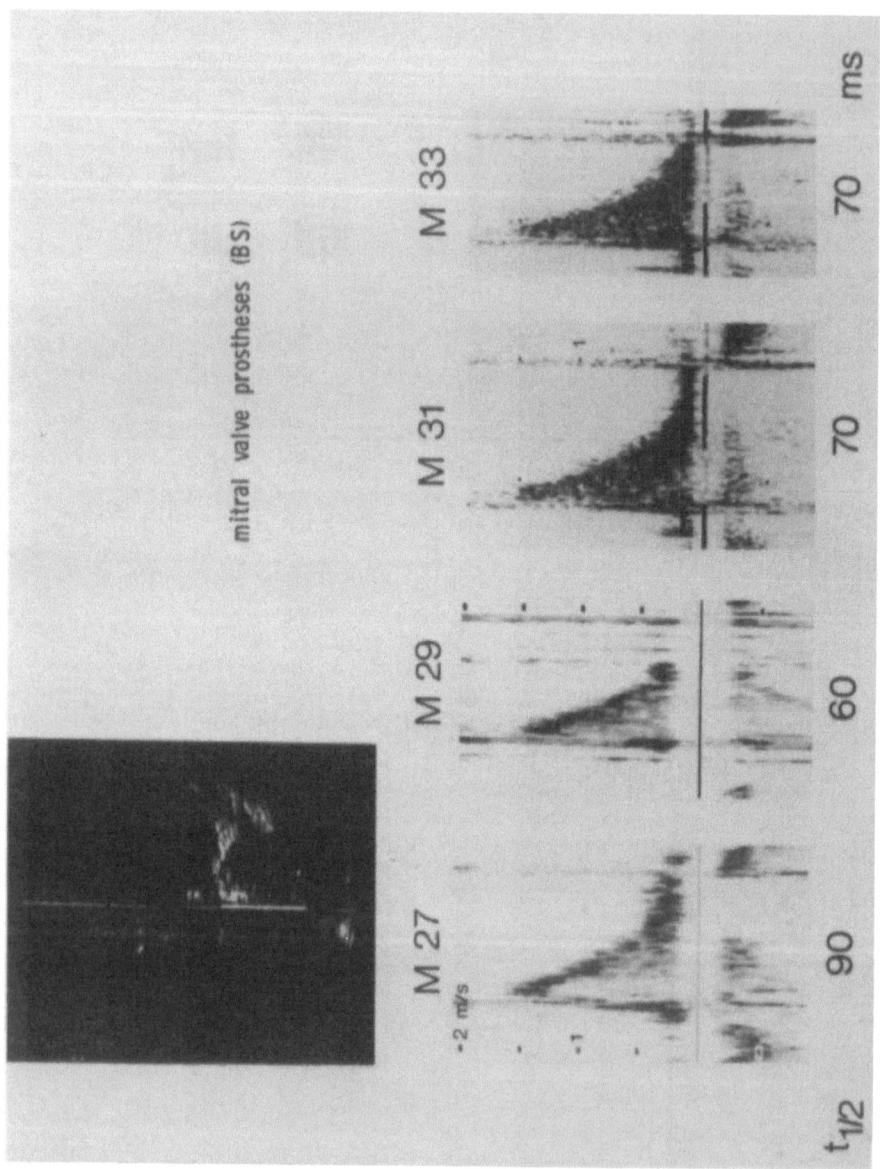

Figure 5. The velocity profile of mitral flow across Björk-Shiley-prostheses of various sizes (M 27–33) and the calculated pressure half-times ($t_{1/2}$).

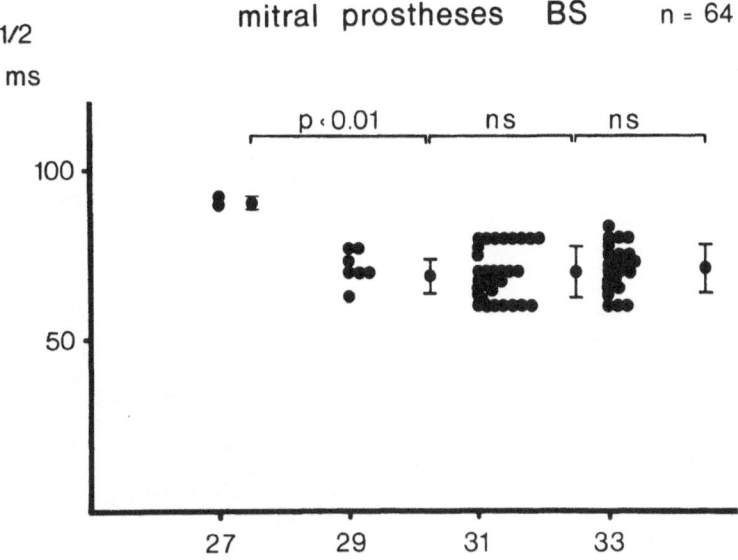

Figure 6. Pressure half-times ($t_{1/2}$) of 64 Björk-Shiley-prostheses (sizes M 27–33) in mitral position including mean values and standard deviations.

Discussion

Our results show that with the aid of Doppler-echocardiography, assessment of mitral valve prostheses can be achieved by non-invasive means.

Using the Bernoulli equation the calculated pressure gradients correlate well with hemodynamic measurements [3, 4] as shown also by other authors [5, 6]. Because of various flow conditions, a certain variability of the data must be expected.

The pressure half-times, used as a measure for the orifice area was slightly prolonged as compared with those in native valves [6] in accordance with the inherent obstruction in valve prostheses. In mechanical prostheses, for each size a low variability of data was found and accordingly to equal orifice areas for M 29–33, the pressure half-times for these sizes showed no statistically significant difference. The somewhat longer pressure half-time for the M 27 is consistent with a smaller orifice area.

For the bioprostheses a tendential decrease in the pressure half-time with increasing size was found. There was, however, a substantial overlap between M 29–35 such that the mean values for the entire groups were statistically not different. Theses results are in good agreement with hemodynamic measurements of valve orifice areas, which showed as well a substantial overlap of the data [7, 8, 9]. This is most probably attributable to the variability of the manufactured products.

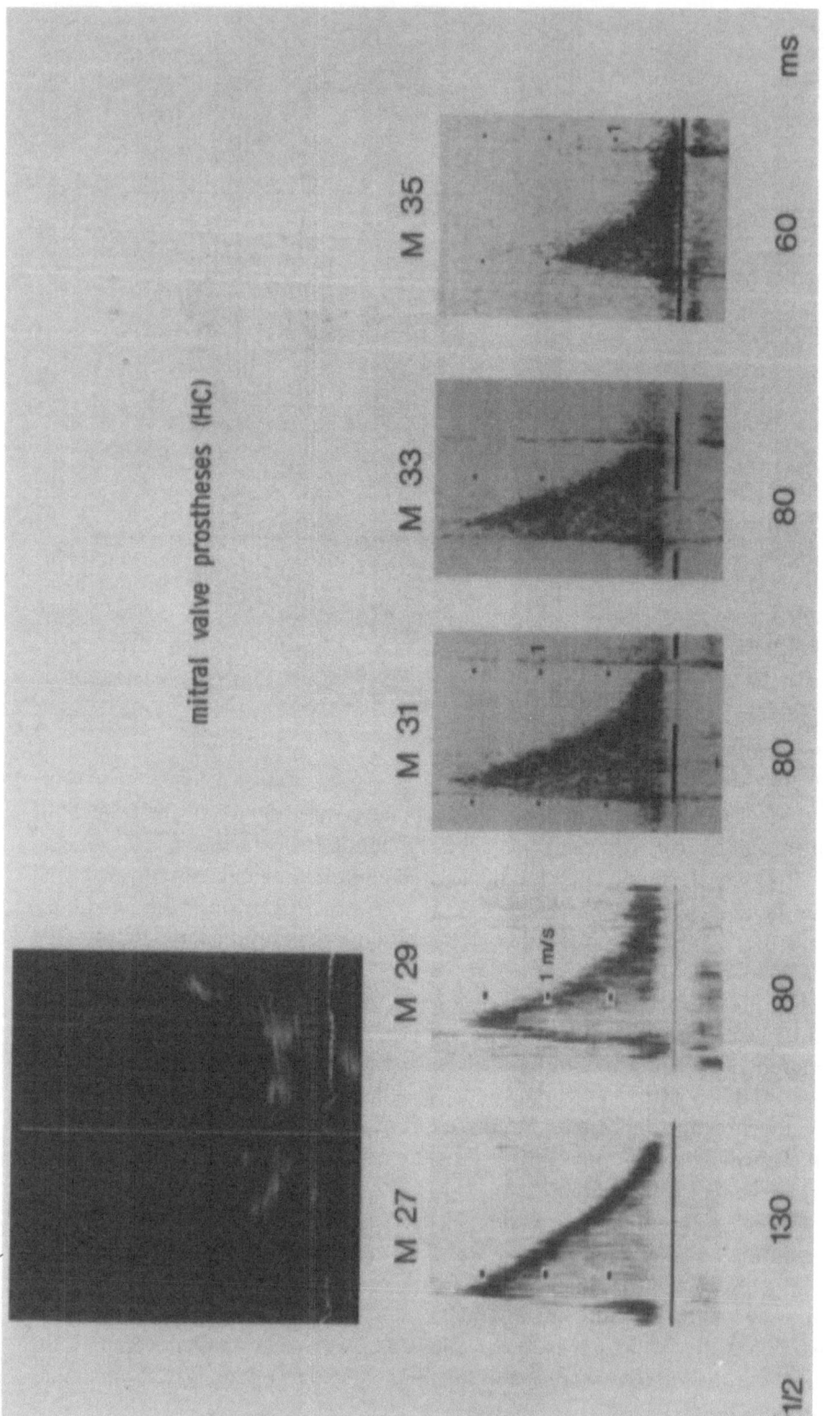

Figure 7. Doppler signals of mitral flow across Hancock-bioprostheses of various sizes (M 27–35). Below the calculated pressure half-times ($t_{1/2}$) are listed.

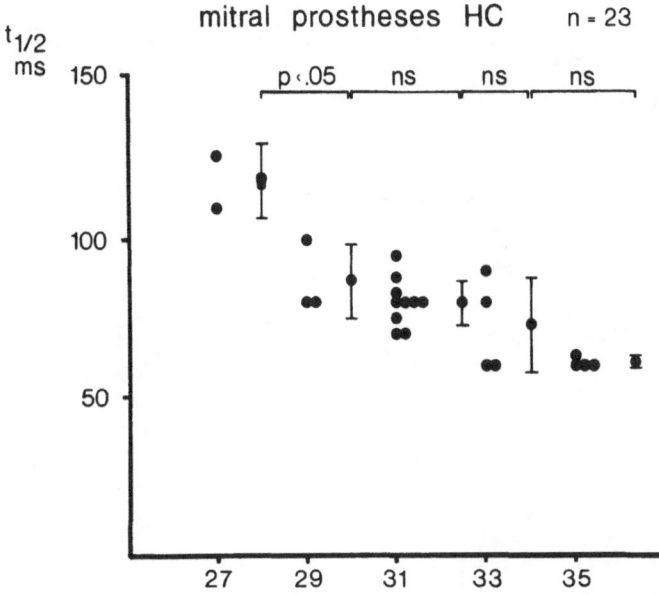

Figure 8. Pressure half-times ($t_{1/2}$) of 23 Hancock-bioprostheses of various sizes (M 27–35) in mitral position with mean values and standard deviations.

Accordingly, the assessment of mechanical prostheses can be based on normal values, whereas, for bioprostheses, follow-up should be referenced to values obtained immediately postoperatively.

Obstruction can be detected and assessed by the prolonged pressure half-time and increased pressure gradient as shown in the examples above. Regurgitation can be detected directly, which might be easier in biological than in mechanical prostheses [6]. Quantification, with respect to the criteria for mitral regurgitation [10, 11], may also be established.

Thus, Doppler echocardiography provides an important improvement in the non-invasive techniques for the assessment of mitral valve prostheses.

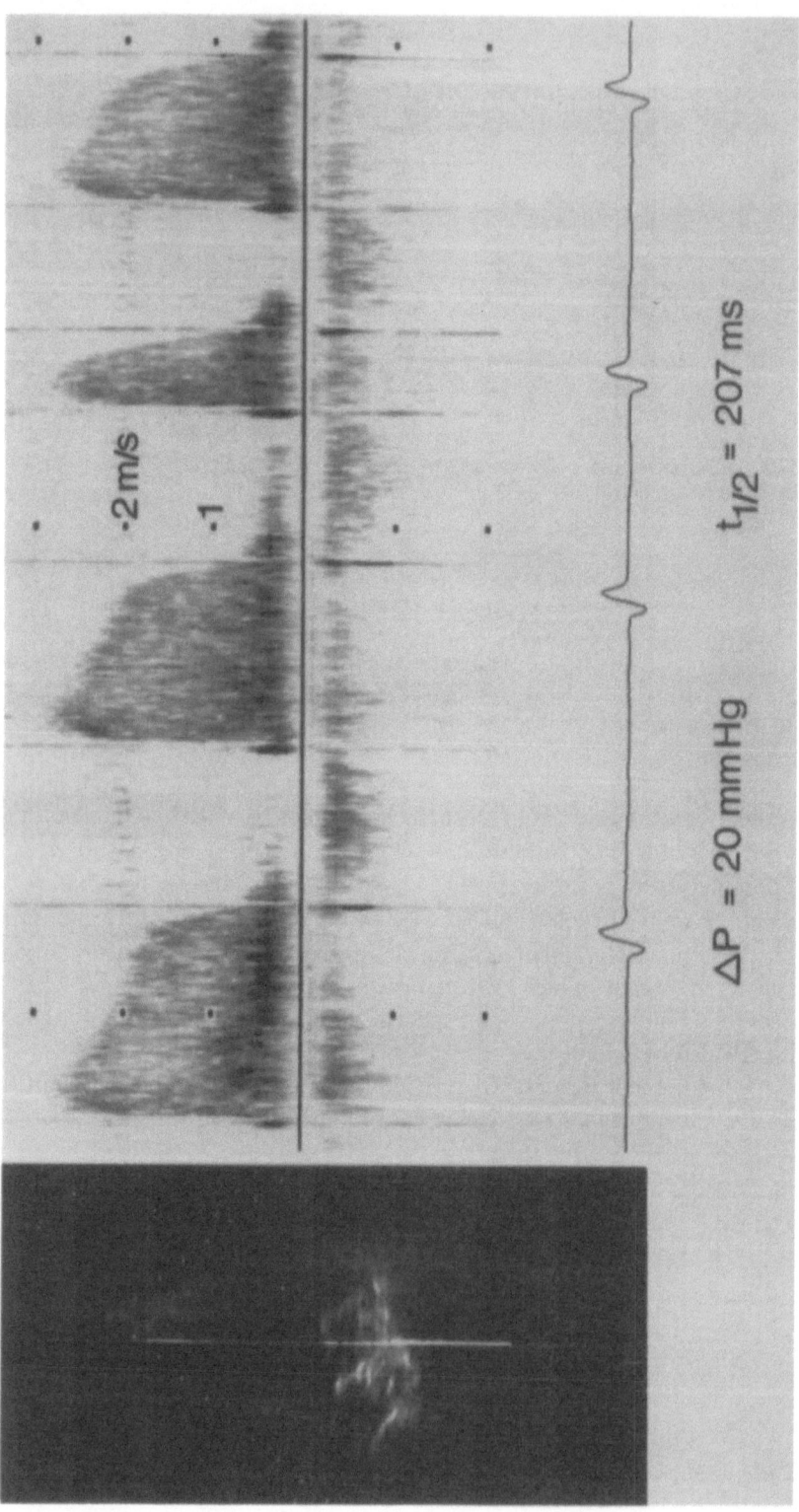

Figure 9. Velocity profile of mitral flow across a stenotic Hancock-bioprosthesis (M 33); note the substantially increased diastolic velocities and the tl at decrease from the early diastolic peak. which leads to a calculated mean diastolic pressure gradient of 20 mmHg and a pressure half-time of 207 ms.

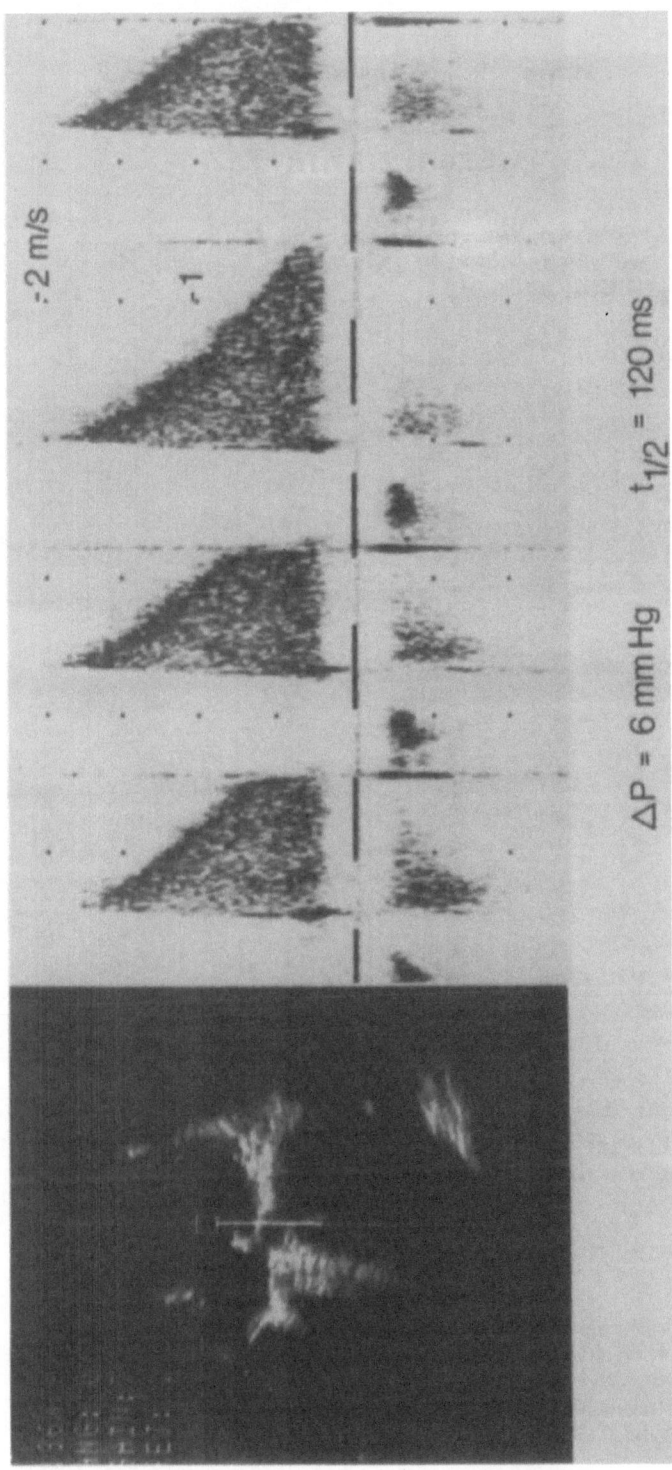

Figure 10. Doppler signal of mitral flow across a slightly stenosic Björk-Shiley-prosthesis (M 27). The mean diastolic pressure gradient was calculated at 6 mmHg; the pressure half-time, at 120 ms, is only slightly prolonged.

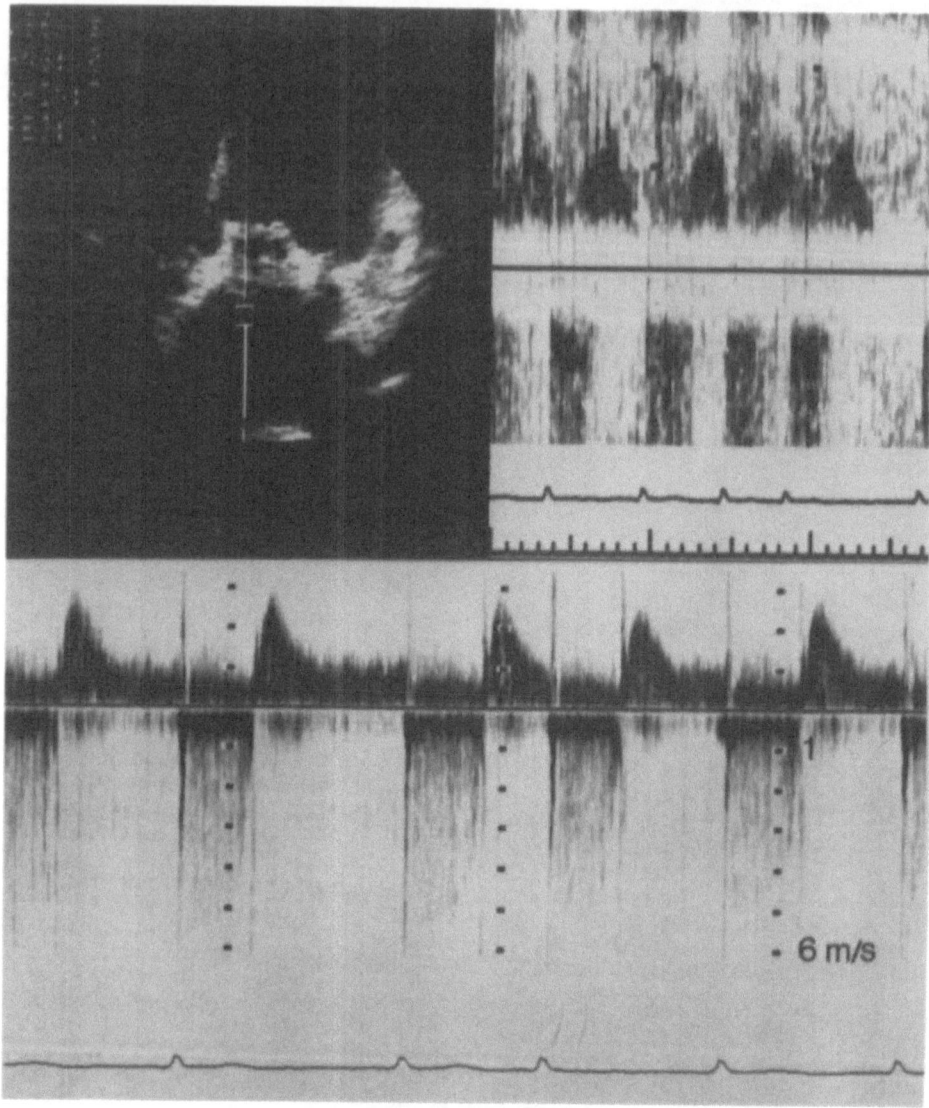

Figure 11. In the upper panel the pulsed Doppler signal proximal to an insufficient mitral prosthesis (Hancock M 35) in the left atrium is demonstrated. The regurgitation can be recognized as a systolic aliasing phenomenon. Below, the velocity profile detected by continuous wave Doppler is shown, whereby the systolic regurgitation jet as well as the increased diastolic velocities can be seen. The decrease of the velocity curve from the early diastolic peak is not prolonged.

References

1. Hatle L, Brubakk A, Tromsdal A, Angelsen B: Noninvasive assessment of pressure drop in mitral stenosis by Doppler ultrasound. Br Heart J 40: 131–140, 1978.
2. Hatle L, Angelsen B,Tromsdal A: Noninvasive assessment of atrioventricular pressure half-time by Doppler ultrasound. Circulation 60: 1096–1104, 1979.
3. Levine FH, Carter JE, Buckley MJ, Daggett WM, Akins CW, Austen WG: Hemodynamic evaluation of Hancock and Carpentier-Edwards bioprostheses. Circulation 64, (II): 192–195, 1981.
4. Bruss KH, Reul H, van Gilse J, Knott E: Pressure drop and velocity fields at four mechanical heart valve prostheses: Björk-Shiley standard, Björk-Shiley concave/convex, Hall-Kaster and St. Jude Medical. Life Support Systems 1: 3–22, 1983.
5. Holen J, Simonsen S, Frøysaker T: An ultrasound Doppler technique for the noninvasive determination of the pressure gradient in the Björk-Shiley mitral valve. Circulation 59: 436–442, 1979.
6. Hatle L, Angelsen B: Doppler ultrasound in Cardiology. Physical Principles and Clinical Applications (2nd ed.). Philadelphia: Lea & Febiger, 1985.
7. Ubago JL, Figueroa A, Colman T, Ochoteco A, Duran CG: Hemodynamic factors that affect calculated orifice areas in the mitral Hancock xenograft valve. Circulation 61: 388–394, 1980.
8. Wright JTM: In vitro comparison between the hydrodynamic characteristics of the Hancock 250 (modified orifice) xenografts and the Björk-Shiley aortic valve prosthesis. Tran. Am. Soc. Artif. Intern. Organs 13: 89–96, 1977.
9. Walker DK, Scotten LN, Modi VJ, Brownlee RT: In vitro assessment of mitral valve prostheses. J. Thorac. Cardiovasc. Surg. 79: 680–688, 1980.
10. Abbasi AS, Allen MW, DeChristofaro D, Ungar J: Detection and estimation of the degree of mitral regurgitation by range-gated pulsed Doppler echocardiography. Circulation 61: 143–147, 1980.
11. Nichol PM, Boughner DR, Persaud JA: Noninvasive assessment of mitral regurgitation by transcutaneous Doppler ultrasound. Circulation 54: 656–661, 1976.

The impact of Doppler in paediatric cardiology

George R. Sutherland and Frances J. Soul

Introduction

The introduction of high resolution cross sectional imaging was the major advance in Paediatric Cardiology of the late '70s. Complex abnormalities of cardiac structure could easily be identified allowing a significant number of infants and children to be referred for surgery on non-invasive grounds alone. However, reliance on imaging alone had its problems. Cross sectional imaging is a superb technique for demonstrating cardiac morphology but cannot give direct haemodynamic information. Any assessment of cardiac haemodynamics had to be indirect and based on clinical examination allied to inferences drawn from the cross sectional images. The presence of valve or subvalve stenosis could be inferred from the images but the severity of the lesion would not be accurately assessed. A moderate or large VSD could be visualised but a limited amount of information could be derived with certainty about its haemodynamics. These are only some of the instances in which imaging was limited in its ability to give a complete non-invasive assessment of cardiac disease. Most of these problems have subsequently been solved by the integration of continuous wave and pulsed Doppler into paediatric imaging systems. With the appropriate use of duplex scanning a precise morphologic and haemodynamic diagnosis can be achieved in virtually every child presenting with congenital heart disease. This can and should lead to more and more children being referred for surgery on non-invasive grounds alone, thus avoiding potentially hazardous cardiac catheterisation.

Both continuous wave and pulsed Doppler are essential to the paediatric cardiologist. Continuous wave, with its ability to resolve high velocities, is essential in the assessment of lesions which produce high velocity jets, e.g.

1. outflow tract stenosis (both severity and type),
2. ventricular septal defects,
3. coarctations.

Pulsed Doppler is essential to

1. the accurate determination of low velocity flow profiles,
2. the assessment of abnormal flow patterns and
3. the accurate assessment of intracardiac shunting where abnormal flow occurs.

No equipment can be considered adequate without both Doppler modalities.

Within the limited space of a book chapter it is impossible to cover all aspects of the role of Doppler in Paediatric Cardiology. Thus the subject has been divided into a number of major sub sections which cover each of the important lesions.

Integration of the information contained in each sub section should allow the investigator to plan and interpret the type of Doppler study required to assess accurately each component of a complex cardiac lesion.

Ventricular septal defects

Both pulsed and continuous wave Doppler are essential to a full study of any ventricular septal defect (VSD) [1, 2]. Each Doppler mode makes its own specific contribution to the assessment of VSD haemodynamics. Whereas imaging will visualise and, thus, classify the morphology of the great majority of moderate or large defects (but normally fails to visualise defects less than 3 mm in diameter) continuous wave Doppler will consistently predict that a defect is present, (if the defect is restrictive) and pulsed Doppler will frequently localise the exit point of the trans-septal jet into the right ventricular cavity. However, both Doppler modalities can provide much more haemodynamic information than simply confirming the presence or absence of a VSD. Let us then consider the information which can be obtained from each.

Continuous wave Doppler (CW) in isolated restrictive VSDs

CW Doppler diagnosis of a VSD relies on the identification of an abnormal pattern of blood flow across the interventricular septum directed towards the Doppler transducer. This flow pattern normally comprises a systolic jet, but frequently, low velocity diastolic flow is also recorded. Where ventricular peak systolic pressures are almost equal the jet velocity exiting across the septum may be as low as 1.5 m/second and in small defects may achieve up to 5 m/second. The pure jet envelope is normally best detected with the transducer in the precordial position at the mid left sternal edge, but the examiner may have to search both high precordial, axillary, apical or subcostal positions to achieve the best alignment to the jet and, hence, the complete jet envelope. In our experience, where ventricular peak systolic pressures are dissimilar CW Doppler will identify a flow disturbance in the right ventricle diagnostic of a VSD in 96% of cases where such a defect is present. In the same study, involving 104 children with VSDs, pulsed Doppler identified the flow disturbance in only 61% of cases confirming its much lower sensitivity. Thus CW Doppler is the technique to use when attempting to identify or exclude a restrictive VSD.

Having identified the presence of a defect and also achieved a complete wave form (Fig. 1), it is possible to determine with reasonable accuracy the peak systolic pressure in the right ventricle [3]. To do this the right arm blood pressure should be measured either before or after the evaluation of the VSD jet by CW Doppler. If CW Doppler confirms normal flow patterns in both the left ventricular outflow tract and ascending aorta then the systolic pressure measured in the

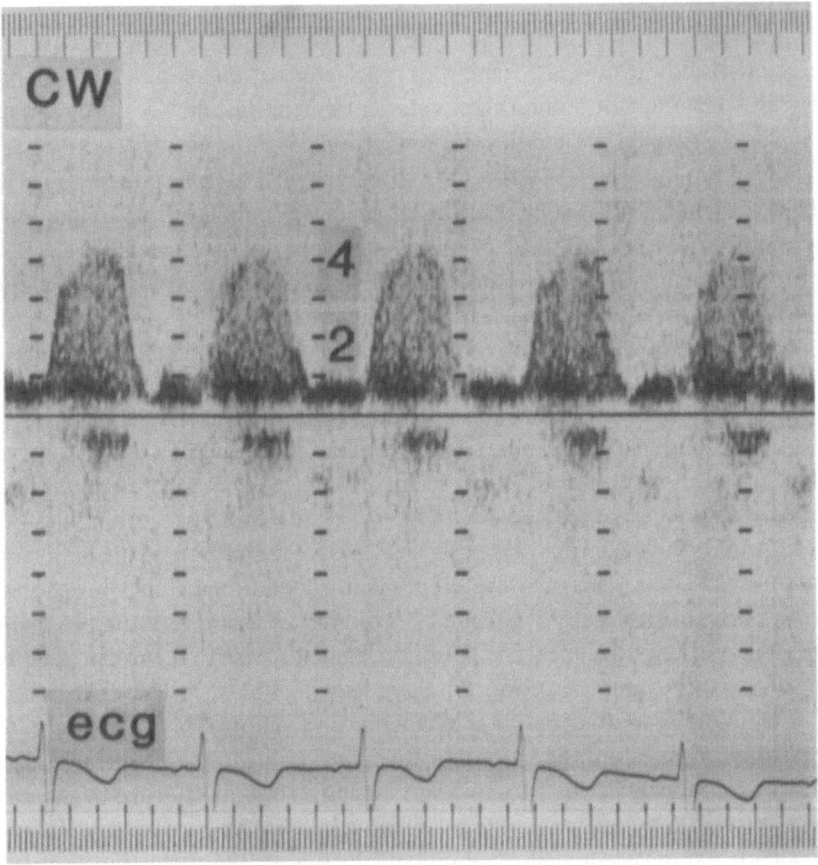

Figure 1. Perimembranous ventricular septal defect – characteristic systolic and diastolic flow patterns recorded using continuous wave Doppler. The systolic jet velocity = 4.3 m/second indicating a transseptal gradient of, at least, 70 mmHg. Note the flow in diastole.

right arm can be assumed to represent left ventricular peak systolic pressure. Using the modified Bernoulli equation ($p_1 - p_2 = 4V^2$) the pressure drop across the septum can be estimated by using the peak velocity of the trans-septal jet. Subtraction of the calculated trans-septal pressure drop from the left ventricular peak systolic pressure should then give an accurate estimate of right ventricular peak systolic pressure. Both the studies of Hatle and ourselves have confirmed the reliability of this estimation where a clear cut VSD jet envelope is obtained. However, it is impossible to obtain a satisfactory envelope in a significant number of patients for one of two reasons:

1. in a small number of patients it is impossible to achieve satisfactory alignment to the jet due to a lack of a suitable echocardiographic window, or
2. there is only turbulent flow and no true jet. This 'spray' like effect into right ventricular cavity is characteristic of very small defects.

In our series of 104 patients with VSDs in whom CW Doppler identified a characteristic flow disturbance in 96%, a satisfactory jet envelope was obtained in only 75%. Having determined right ventricular peak systolic pressure, and also having demonstrated normal flow velocities in the right ventricular outflow tract and main pulmonary artery, it is correct to assume peak systolic pulmonary artery pressure = peak systolic right ventricular pressure (mmHg). The estimation of pulmonary artery peak systolic pressure in the clinical assessment of a VSD is important information, both in context of the risks of pulmonary vascular disease and the demonstration of reduction in defect size.

It is relatively common to observe a sequential increase in VSD jet velocity as an indicator of partial defect closure in an infant with an isolated VSD before any clinical or echocardiographic changes are noted. As right ventricular peak systolic pressure evaluation is such an important estimation it would be useful to have a second method of determining this. In theory this may be done by determining the peak systolic pressure drop across the tricuspid valve by recording the peak velocity of the physiological tricuspid incompetence jet (present in the majority of paediatric patients). This pressure drop, when added to the clinically estimated venous pressure (normally 7–10 mmHg) will give an accurate estimate of right ventricular peak systolic pressure. Unfortunately it is rare to record an adequate tricuspid incompetence wave form in patients with VSDs. In 104 VSDs studied with CW Doppler a full tricuspid incompetence wave form was only recorded in 4% of cases. Our failure to record this wave form is due to the practical problem of having to interrogate the tricuspid valve using a continuous wave beam which passes through the right ventricle in which turbulence exists due to a VSD jet. Our experience suggests it is very difficult to find a transducer position from which the tricuspid incompetence jet may be separated from the VSD jet. This problem is especially difficult in perimembranous defects. It may only be resolved by the use of integrated duplex/high pulse repetition frequency pulsed Doppler which should, by sampling the right atrial floor, accurately resolve the tricuspid regurgitation jet without interference from the VSD jet.

Continuous wave Doppler (CW) in unrestricted defects

Hatle has stated that no VSD flow signals are recorded from children and adults with large VSDs in which the peak systolic right and left ventricular pressures are equal. This would be expected as no apparent pressure exists to give a Doppler signal. Such defects will normally be easily visualised on cross sectional imaging. However, our experience has indicated that this is not always the case. In a high proportion of unrestrictive defects low velocity flow (<1.5 m/second) can be recorded across the defect which may alter in direction up to four times during the cardiac cycle with both left to right and right to left shunting components. These flow patterns are best recorded on pulsed Doppler with the sample volume placed in the defect but may also be recorded by the experienced examiner using continuous wave. They are observed both in patients with Eisenmenger VSD and patients where an unrestrictive VSD is part of a complex heart malformation, e.g. Tetralogy of Fallot.

Pulsed Doppler – restrictive defects

As indicated above, an important role of pulsed Doppler in the assessment of VSDs is to determine the site of the defect. This is normally carried out by interrrogating the right ventricular aspect of the ventricular septum in a number of planes to determine the exit point of the VSD jet into the right ventricle. The pulsed Doppler available on most systems will normally alias at approximately 3 to 4 m/second and thus is only capable of resolving low velocity VSD jets. High pulse repetition frequency Doppler can resolve jets of 5–6 m/second and potentially can accurately evaluate right heart systolic pressures. However, as indicated above, CW Doppler provides both a more sensitive and more accurate method of deriving this information.

Potentially with pulsed Doppler it should be possible to identify the exit points of two or more VSDs, if multiple defects are present. Although more than one defect can, on occasion, be identified, the relative insensitivity of the technique allied to the presence of widespread flow disturbance in the right ventricle means that little reliance can be placed on a pulsed Doppler examination excluding the presence of a second VSD. (CW Doppler is of no value in this regard.)

Pulsed Doppler in the assessment of Qp : Qs in VSDs

Perhaps the most important role of pulsed Doppler in the assessment of VSDs is, in its theoretical ability to determine the magnitude of the associated intracardiac shunting [4]. By recording both the flow profiles and vessel diameter from both pulmonary artery and ascending aorta it is theoretically possible to calculate Qp : Qs with an accuracy theoretically not possible with CW Doppler. A series of papers have reported excellent correlations between Qp : Qs derived from simultaneous pulsed Doppler/imaging studies when compared to the results calculated at cardiac catheterisation. These studies have in the most part been carried out in older children with relatively trivial intracardiac shunts. Our experience has differed considerably from these studies. Major problems arose in determining the pulmonary artery diameter. In the critical age group (i.e. children <2 years of age) the pulmonary artery is a distensible structure which may vary up to 35% in diameter during one cardiac cycle. As the flow calculation requires the diameter measured to be squared (flow = cross section area × mean velocity) then this automatically introduces a significant error. Furthermore, the flow profile in the pulmonary artery may not be flat. The flow estimation may be further complicated by the occurrence of turbulent flow in the pulmonary artery often associated with high flow VSDs. Both these latter two factors may further add to the inaccuracy of pulmonary flow estimation. In our experience, Qp : Qs calculation by integrated imaging and Doppler is consistently accurate only in the older child (i.e. >2 years) with a small or moderate shunt. It would appear to be an inaccurated measurement in a significant number of children under 2 years – precisely the age group in which the estimation is of most value. Other methods of estimating Qp : Qs such as comparing flow across the mitral and aortic valves have their own major technical limitations and may be equally inaccurate. Perhaps the main value of pulmonary artery flow estimation by pulsed Doppler is in comparing serial flow evaluations in the same patient when attempting to determine the natural history of a VSD. In this context a progressive fall in the peak systolic velocity in the pulmonary artery towards normal values is invariably related to either a reduction in pulmonary blood flow, and hence intracardiac shunting, or to an increase in pulmonary vascular resistance.

Atrial septal defects

Defects in the atrial septum are of 4 differing types each with a different position in the septum and each with a unique spectrum of associated cardiac abnormalities:

1. secundum defects,
2. sinus venosus defects,

3. coronary sinus defects and
4. primum (partial atrioventricular) defects.

Whereas cross sectional imaging is essential to the correct morphologic diagnosis of each type, Doppler is essential both to the evaluation of the associated hemodynamic disturbances and, thus, the confirmation of the diagnosis. Using imaging alone, areas of echo 'drop out' may be identified within the atrial septal echo. The majority of these will represent true atrial septal defects (ASD) but a significant number will be false positive findings. These 'false positive' areas of echo drop out occur most commonly in two sites:

1. in the region of the foramen ovale where the septum is very thin but present and
2. in the superior portion of the atrial septum where resolution may be poor.

Pulsed Doppler should be used to determine if an area of atrial septal drop out represents a defect [5]. Initially the sample volume should be placed on the right atrial surface of the defect and aligned as near parallel to flow as possible. This normally is best effected by imaging the atrial septum from either a low parasternal or subcostal position. Where predominantly left to right shunting exists across the defect a characteristic flow pattern will readily be detected (Fig. 2). Flow will normally commence in early to mid systole and achieve a peak velocity in late systole. A second period of left to right flow is normally observed following atrial contraction. Flow reversal (i.e. right to left shunting) is often seen in late diastole spilling over into early systole. The above flow patterns are characteristic of both secundum and sinus venosus defects. Coronary sinus defects pose different problems as pulsed Doppler will record coronary sinus flow as left to right flow near the floor of the right atrium originating from the posterior aspect of the atrial septum in the majority of normal children with an intact atrial septum. Coronary sinus defects are difficult to image but should be suspected when three factors are present:

1. a persisting left superior vena cava,
2. an area of septal 'drop out' associated with the coronary sinus and
3. increased velocity of coronary sinus flow.

Partial atrioventricular defects provide an even more complex challenge. Imaging will predict the precise anatomy. However, morphologic assessment alone has its limitations in clinical assessment, and, equally important is a precise haemodynamic evaluation of each component of the lesion. A combination of pulsed and continuous wave Doppler can be used to evaluate the complex shunting patterns associated within this complex spectrum of defects. Normally a primum defect will demonstrate three main abnormal flow patterns:

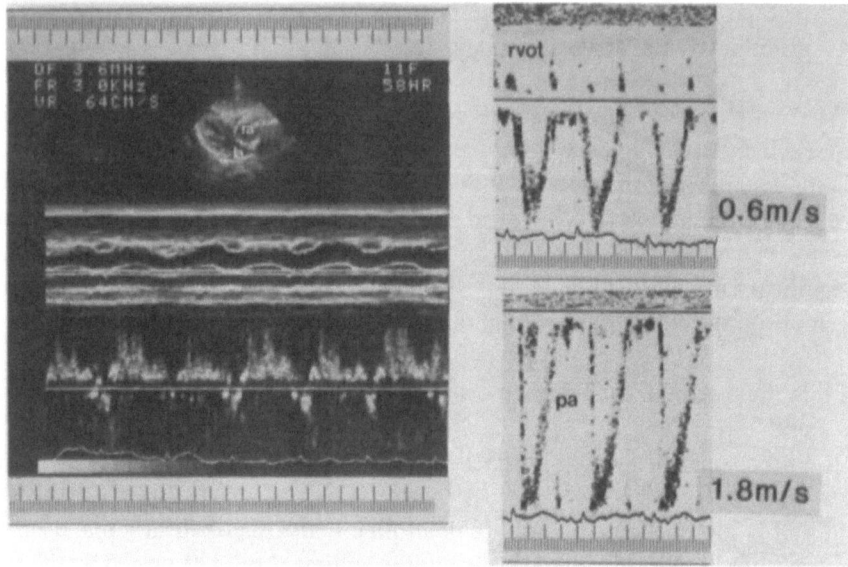

Figure 2. The characteristic flow patterns recorded by a pulsed Doppler study in a child with a secundum atrial septal defect.

Left hand panel: With the sample volume placed at the right hand aspect of the defect flow is seen to pass left to right across the defect, thus, confirming that the area of echo 'drop out' constitutes a defect.

Right upper panel: Normal flow velocity was recorded in the right ventricular outflow tract.

Right lower panel: Characteristically these patients have a small flow gradient across the pulmonary valve. Note the acceleration in flow to 1.8 m/second. This does not represent a structural pulmonary valve abnormality.

1. left to right atrial low velocity flow,
2. a left ventricular to right atrial high velocity jet, and
3. a left ventricular to left atrial high velocity jet of atrioventricular valve incompetence.

Significant incompetence of the right portion of the common valve may also exist, giving a fourth abnormal flow pattern, but this is relatively uncommon. Pulsed Doppler will identify all these flow patterns. It can be used to track the regurgitant jet from the atrioventricular valve into both atrial chambers. Both signal strength and distance of jet extension into the atria can be used to give an approximate evaluation of the degree of valve regurgitation, but it must be emphasised that this may give misleading results even when evaluated by an experienced investigator. Indirect estimation of peak systolic right ventricular pressure from the peak velocity of the tricuspid incompetence jet (normally a reliable method of right ventricular pressure estimation in other types of ASDs) is an unreliable method in partial atrioventricular defects because of the presence of the direct left ventricular to right atrial shunt. Where a high velocity jet is detected in the right atrium there is no method of ascertaining whether this originates in the right or left ventricle.

Pulsed Doppler in the assessment of Qp : Qs in atrial septal defects

Estimation of Qp : Qs in secundum, sinus venosus and coronary sinus defects by a combination of imaging vessel diameter and determining ascending aortic and pulmonary artery flow patterns by pulsed Doppler has proved to be more accurate than the same estimation has proved to be in ventricular septal defects [6, 7, 8]. It should be noted, however, that Qp : Qs is not a constant value in a patient with a secundum defect but may vary significantly both with heart rate and position. Of equal value in determining Qp : Qs is a pulsed Doppler comparison of flow profiles across the tricuspid and mitral valve orifices [9]. Tricuspid peak velocity in the normal child is always less than mitral peak velocity. Where a significant left to right atrial shunt is present, the ratio of the peak velocities across these valves are reversed, the tricuspid peak velocity being the same by one and a half times the mitral peak velocity. Such a reversal confirms the presence of a significant atrial shunt. Where a small left to right atrial shunt exists the tricuspid and mitral peak velocities tend to be the same.

Patent or persistent ductus arteriosus

A patent ductus arteriosus is defined to be a morphologically normal ductus arteriosus which remains patent in a premature infant. The normal mechanisms for duct closure are present and will close the duct spontaneously as the neonate approaches 40 weeks gestation. A persistent duct is morphologically abnormal. It does not have, and never will have, a mechanism whereby complete closure will be effected. Both structures will give rise to identical unique disturbances of flow within the great vessels which are readily identified by Doppler. Imaging can identify a ductus in the great majority of infants but both false positive and false negative diagnoses can be made. Even where a duct is imaged it may be possible to ascertain if there is flow through it using imaging alone. Both continuous wave [12] and pulsed Doppler [10] can be used to determine if ductus flow is present. Sampling flow in the duct will give rise to a continuous pattern of flow (Fig. 3) which rises to peak velocity at end systole. The mid-systolic peak velocity achieved is a direct reflection of the pulmonary artery pressure. The higher the peak velocity achieved the greater the pressure difference between the systemic and pulmonary artery pressure and, hence, the lower the peak systolic pulmonary pressure. Sampling flow in the descending aorta and the head and neck vessels using pulsed Doppler will demonstrate marked diastolic flow reversal in all patients with a moderate or large ductus. [10] Diastolic flow is much less pro-

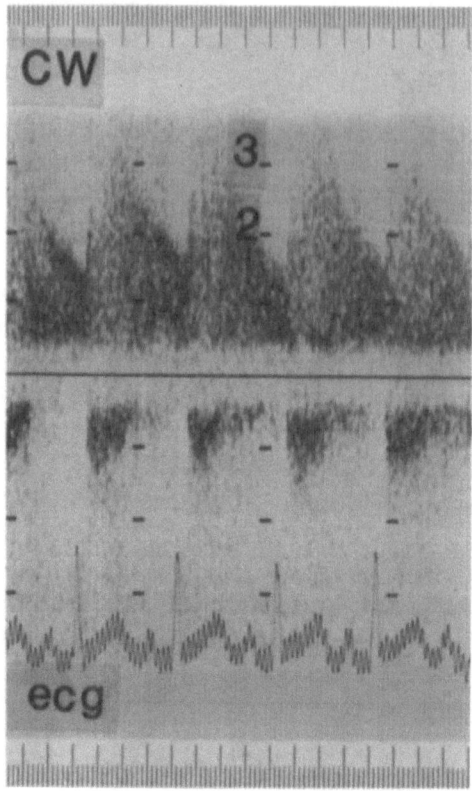

Figure 3. Typical pattern of continuous flow recorded by CW Doppler from a premature infant with a moderate sized PDA. The peak velocity of flow = 3.4 m/second indicating low pulmonary artery pressure.

nounced where left to right duct shunting is small. Sampling flow in the pulmonary artery away from the orifice of the duct using pulsed Doppler will given rise to a number of differing flow patterns. Where pulmonary artery pressure is less than systolic then continuous flow will be recorded throughout the pulmonary arterial tree. Where systemic and pulmonary systolic pressures are equal then systolic flow in the pulmonary artery will be normal with flow from the duct entering the pulmonary artery only in diastole. This diastolic flow will be of low velocity because of the near equal systemic and pulmonary diastolic pressures. In very rare cases (normally in neonates with high pulmonary resistance) the duct may be widely patent but has no measurable flow across it because of identical pressures and resistances in both systemic and pulmonary circulations. In neonates with persistent fetal circulation pulsed Doppler will clearly demonstrate the right to left duct shunting patterns. In our experience, pulsed Doppler has become invaluable in accurately assessing pulmonary haemodynamics in the premature infant.

Other conditions which simulate ductus flow

A Doppler study may demonstrate continuous flow into the pulmonary vessels in other situations. Pulmonary atresia, either with confluent pulmonary arteries supplied by a ductus, or with no true pulmonary artery and lung blood supply via collaterals arising from the descending aorta will demonstrate a continuous flow pattern on pulsed Doppler throughout the pulmonary vascular bed. Again, the higher the peak velocity of this flow, the lower the pulmonary artery pressure. Both aorto-pulmonary shunts and an aorto-pulmonary window will give rise to ductus-type flow patterns as will anomalous coronary arteries arising from the pulmonary artery. The pulmonary artery flow pattern in truncus arteriosus is similar. All these lesions must be differentiated by imaging – Doppler will only identify the characteristic flow disturbance associated with an aorto-pulmonary shunt which is common to them all.

Aortic coarctation in infants and older children

Coarctation of the aorta presents the investigator with very differing problems in the neonate when compared to the lesion in the older infant/child. In the neonatal group the lesion is better termed Coarctation Syndrome as the aortic lesion is frequently complex and takes one of many forms, (e.g. aortic interruption; juxtaductal coarctation plus severe arch hypoplasia, abdominal coarctation etc.). In addition, the coarctation is almost invariably associated with a ductus arteriosus whose calibre and flow patterns vary from the widely patent with a left to right shunt to the extremely stenotic with a right to left shunt. Furthermore, the aortic lesion is often associated with a series of complex intracardiac malformations, e.g. multiple muscular VSDs, left ventricular outflow tract obstruction, mitral valve abnormalities etc. Thus, a comprehensive Doppler study in coarctation syndrome involves a Doppler study of all the flow patterns within the heart and great vessels as well as a full imaging study. Neonatal coarctation syndrome remains one of the most complex non invasive investigations which the Paediatric Cardiologist faces.

Neonatal coarctation syndrome

Unlike the confirmation of the diagnosis of an aortic coarctation in the older patient in whom CW Doppler directed from a suprasternal position will, invariably, (with experience) demonstrate a high velocity jet in the descending aorta (see below) there may be no high velocity jet recorded in a neonate with severe coarctation. Why is this? The key to understanding this lies in the appreciation of the role of the ductus in the neonatal coarctation syndrome. The duct will normally be the agent which maintains flow in the descending aorta below the coarctation, as there are rarely any significant collateral vessels. The neonate is normally pulmonary hypertensive and, thus, near systemic pressure will normally exist in the descending aorta. Thus the jet velocity across the coarctation will rarely be greater than 2.5 m/second. Forward flow is normally restricted to systole and flow reversal is noted in diastole as flow reverses in the descending aorta to flow back into the ductus. A similar pattern is normally found in aortic interruption with a stenotic duct. In this lesion the obligatory right to left shunt across the obstructive duct gives rise to an identical systolic jet in descending aorta. With diastolic flow reversal into the pulmonary artery. In both conditions, where the infant is receiving prostaglandin therapy and the ductus is widely patent then no abnormal systolic jet will be present. Thus although the identification of a systolic jet in the descending aorta is diagnostic of a descending aortic abnormality in a neonate, it does not differentiate a coarctation from aortic interruption. Furthermore, failure to record a high velocity descending aortic jet does not rule out a severe obstructive descending aortic lesion. The diagnosis of aortic arch/descending aortic abnormalities in a neonate remains primarily an imaging diagnosis. Similarly the severity of the intracardiac lesions may be inaccurately assessed by Doppler as the systolic pressure in both ventricles and both great vessels is normally equal. Multiple muscular VSDs can be just as easily missed on Doppler as on imaging. Left ventricular outflow tract obstruction may be underestimated. Mitral stenosis is not accurately assessed in the presence of high left atrial blood flow and raised left ventricular end diastolic pressure.

Isolated aortic coarctation in the older patient

The aortic coarctation found in the older infant and child is remarkably consistent in its morphology. It is normally located in the typical juxtaductal position opposite the origin of the left subclavian. Its structure is 'ring form' and is not associated with any proximal aortic hypoplasia. By a few months of age multiple collateral vessels have usually developed to supply the descending aorta. A co-existing patent ductus is rarely present. The lesion is commonly associated with a bicuspid aortic valve but other intracardiac abnormalities are uncommon.

CW Doppler is the best method of confirming the pressure of this coarctation. With the transducer placed in the suprasternal notch a high velocity jet commencing in systole will be recorded in the descending aorta. The velocity of the jet will increase with the severity of the coarctation as with the duration of the velocity curve. In very severe coarctations descending aortic flow may not commence until almost mid systole and then be prolonged well into diastole. In some severe coarctations flow may continue until the following systole (Fig. 4). This may in part be due to diastolic forward flow in the collateral vessels. In mild coarctations flow is restricted to systole with a peak flow velocity invariably less than 3 m/second.

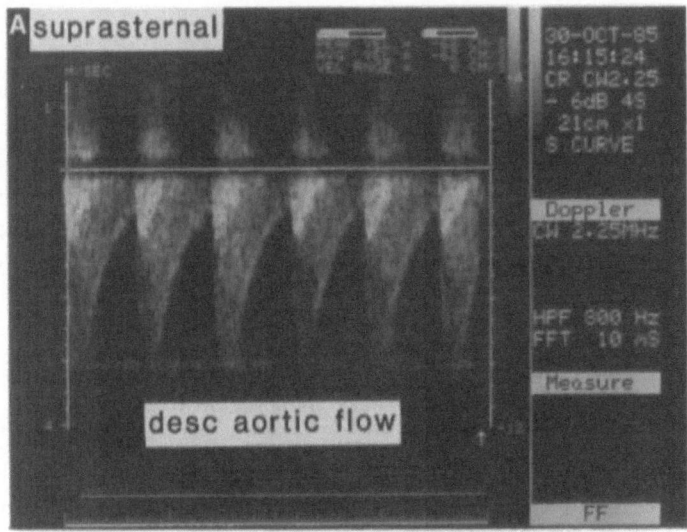

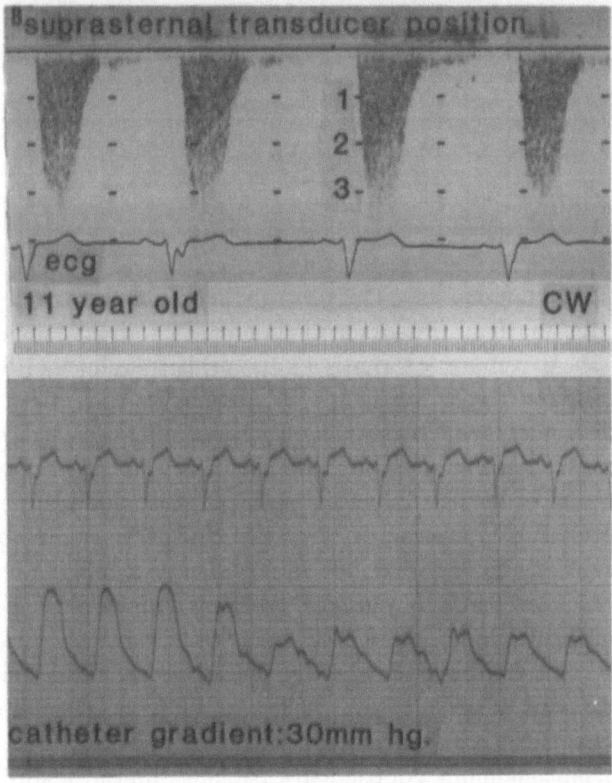

Figure 4. a. Severe coarctation – 4-year-old. From a suprasternal transducer position CW Doppler has identified a high velocity jet in descending aorta = 3.1 m/second. Note the abnormal nature of the flow with prolonged flow occurring across the coarctation in diastole. This pattern is characteristic of a severe coarctation.

Figure 4. b. Moderate coarctation – 11-year-old. Note the differing wave form in this coarctation. Flow across the lesion is confined to systole and there is no significant radio-femoral delay. Despite the same apparent gradient (= 3 m/second) being recorded the lesion is clearly less severe as judged on the CW waveform.

Outflow tract stenosis

Stenosis of either the right or left ventricular outflow tracts is a common finding in paediatric cardiology. It may present as either an isolated lesion, or may be part of a more complex abnormality. Frequently the obstruction is complex with both valve and subvalve stenosis co-existing. Subvalve stenosis itself may be equally complex being

1. multilevel, and
2. possessing elements of both fixed and dynamic obstruction.

Cross sectional imaging will identify the morphology of obstructive lesions within an outflow tract, but cannot accurately assess either its severity or determine the relative value of each component where the obstruction is multilevel. A combination of continuous wave and pulsed Doppler can largely solve these problems.

Semilunar valve stenosis

Imaging will frequently identify a semilunar valve as being stenotic by visualising a combination of thickened valve leaflets, restricted cusp motion or systolic 'doming' of the valve. However, imaging is limited in its ability to predict the valve gradient. Continuous wave Doppler, has proved to be extremely accurate in measuring the maximal instantaneous gradient across a stenotic semilunar valve in children. Valvar aortic stenosis is normally best evaluated from an apical transducer position with the beam aligned to ascending aortic flow. The trans-valve flow will be recorded with certainty only when the valve clicks are simultaneously recorded with the flow profile. The high velocity jet of aortic valve stenosis is easily recorded in children and with due care should never be missed. In every case of aortic stenosis, an attempt should also be made to obtain the jet waveform from both the subcostal and suprasternal positions as a check on the maximal jet velocity. Similarly pulsed Doppler examination of the subaortic region should be carried out in every case to exclude subvalve stenosis, and to check that the velocity of blood flow below the aortic valve is normal. The flow profile recorded from a patient with isolated valvar aortic stenosis is that of a 'fixed' obstruction (Fig. 5) in which the maximal jet velocity occurs early in systole. In a significant number of paediatric patients with valvar aortic stenosis a pulsed Doppler examination of the subvalve region will demonstrate a second co-existing 'dynamic' obstruction waveform with a much lower peak velocity which rises to a peak in late systole (Fig. 6).

Immediately following successful aortic valvotomy this secondary subvalve obstruction may temporarily become much more marked with Doppler recording a dynamic obstruction waveform with a peak velocity of >4 m/second, (Fig. 7).

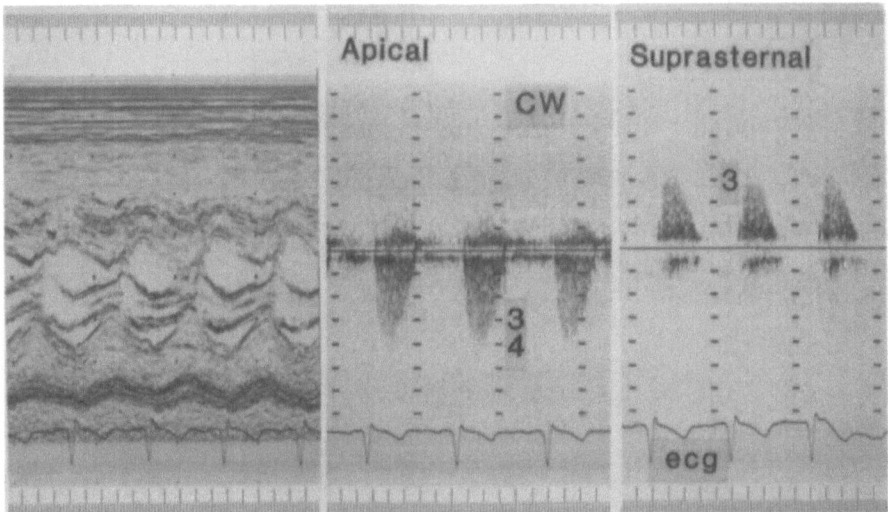

Figure 5. Isolated valvar aortic stenosis in a 3-year-old.

Left hand panel: M-mode echo demonstrating concentric left ventricular hypertrophy.

Middle panel: The characteristic 'fixed obstruction' jet of 3.7 m/second obtained by placing the CW transducer at the apex. The maximal instantaneous gradient derived from the modified Bernoulli equation = 55 mmHg.

Right hand panel: The high velocity jet has also been recorded by placing the CW transducer in the suprasternal position. Jet velocity recorded from this position is lower at 3.2 m/second and the jet envelope less clear. This is due to failure to align the CW beam to the jet from the suprasternal position.

This post operative dynamic obstruction waveform will normally be reduced or abolished in the short term by a combination of volume supplements and Verapamil (or Beta-blockade), and will subsequently regress in time, if the valve stenosis has been effectively relieved.

Valvar pulmonary stenosis is normally best evaluated with the transducer directed towards the pulmonary valve from the subcostal position. As with the aortic valve, other precordial transducer positions should be used to make certain that correct alignment to the jet has been achieved. Normally the highest jet velocity will be recorded from the subcostal position. As with aortic stenosis, the waveform of isolated pulmonary stenosis is that of a fixed obstruction. Calculation of the maximal instantaneous gradient derived by using the modified Bernoulli equation has been shown to be remarkably accurate in a number of simultaneous Doppler/catheter studies. Pulsed Doppler examination of the right ventricular outflow tract will reveal a secondary, low velocity, 'dynamic' obstruction waveform below the stenotic pulmonary valve in almost every case. As with aortic stenosis, pulmonary valvotomy may result in an immediate reduction in the 'fixed' obstruction, but an associated dramatic increase in the subvalve dynamic obstruction. The management of this is the same as for the post aortic valvotomy patient (see above).

198

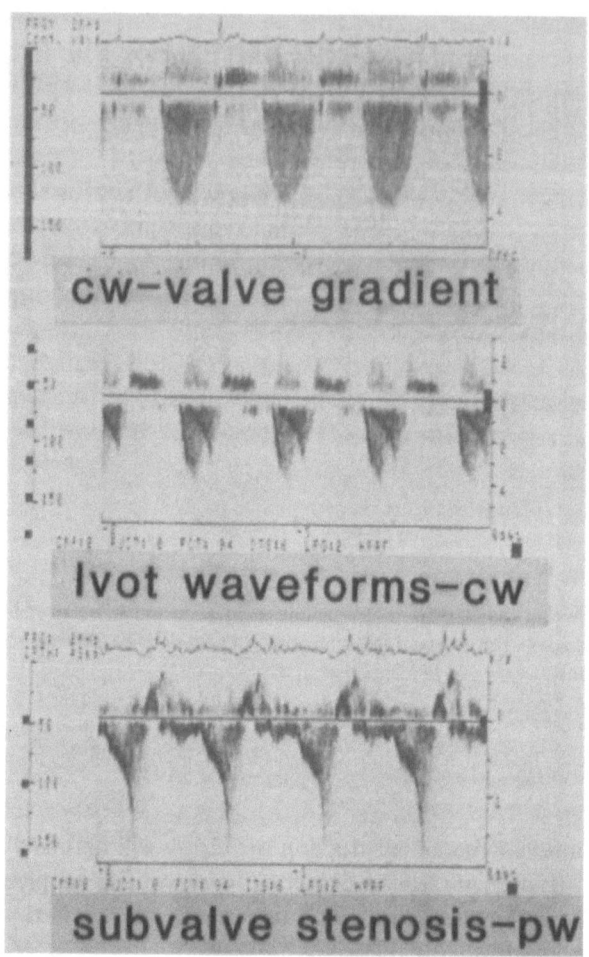

Figure 6. Co-existing aortic valvar and subvalve obstruction – 9-year-old.
Upper panel: CW Doppler – apical transducer position. A waveform indicating a fixed obstruction with a peak velocity of 3.2 m/second, was recorded across the aortic valve.
Middle panel: CW Doppler – angulation of the transducer to interrogate the subvalve area produced two superimposed waveforms: 1. the fixed obstruction waveform of the valve stenosis, and 2. a slow rising dynamic waveform indicating a secondary subvalve dynamic obstruction.
Lower panel: High PRF Doppler – pulsed Doppler analysis of the left ventricular outflow tract confirmed the dynamic obstruction to be at subvalve level – peak velocity = 3.8 m/second.

Great care must be taken in interpreting the gradient calculated by Doppler in patients in whom severe isolated semilunar valve stenosis is associated with severe malfunction of the underlying ventricle. In some neonates where critical aortic stenosis has caused severe left ventricular dysfunction the trans-valve gradient may be misleadingly low at <2 m/second. In such patients treatment with an inotropic agent will normally temporarily improve ventricular function

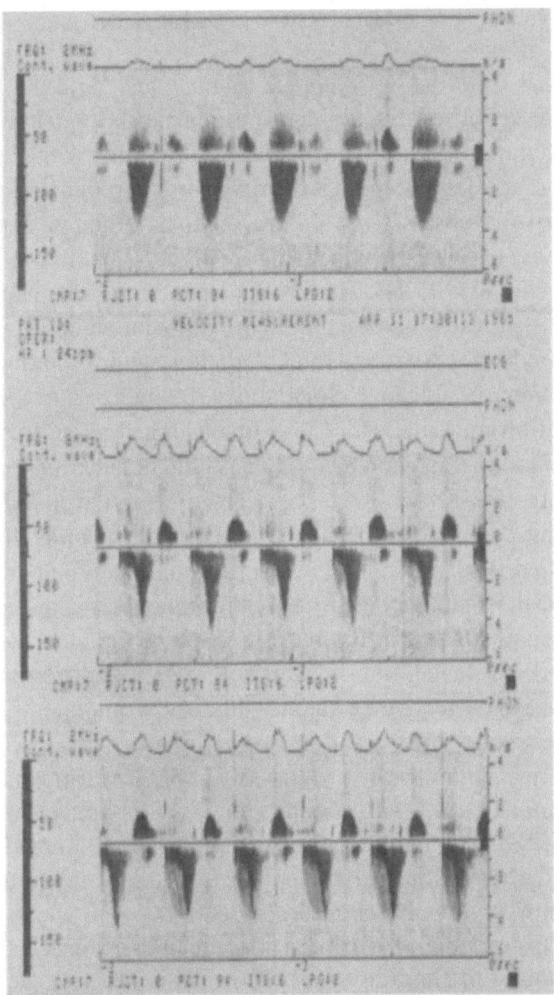

Figure 7. Post-operative study – Critical aortic stenosis of a 5-day-old neonate – post-valvotomy. The pre-operative Doppler gradient was >100 mmHg. No subvalve dynamic gradient had been recorded. The 1 hour post-operative continuous wave study demonstrated a residual fixed obstruction at valve level of some 40 mmHg *(upper panel)*. Continuous wave assessment of the subvalve area demonstrated two superimposed wave forms *(middle panel)*: 1. the slow rising waveform indicative of dynamic subvalve obstruction with a late systolic peak velocity of 4.2 m/second, and 2. the waveform of mitral regurgitation. In the *lower panel* the transducer has been angled towards the mitral orifice and the full mitral regurgitation waveform recorded with the dynamic subvalve obstruction waveform still superimposed.

and, as a consequence, increase the trans-valve gradient to >4 m/second, allowing confirmation of the diagnosis. Similar care must be taken in assessing the trans-valve gradient in neonates with critical pulmonary stenosis and severe right ventricular dysfunction. Again, inotrope infusion will increase the gradient and confirm the diagnosis.

Subvalve stenosis

Subvalvar stenosis is normally a complex lesion which varies in its morphology depending on which outflow tract is involved. The most frequent form of isolated subvalve obstruction in the left ventricular outflow tract is the subaortic fibromuscular membrane. Less common is the fibromuscular tunnel. Least common is childhood hypertropic obstructive cardiomyopathy. Although, in theory, each of these may occur as an isolated lesion, components of each often occur in combination forming a complex lesion. Within the right ventricular outflow tract the common form of subvalve obstruction is infundibular stenosis – in infants this tends to be a predominantly dynamic obstruction with a relatively small fixed component. In time the dynamic element is virtually lost and the outflow tract becomes a long fibromuscular tunnel creating a long segment fixed obstruction.

In theory the modified Bernoulli equation should not give an accurate gradient assessment where an obstruction is long segment, multilevel and contains both fixed and dynamic components. Despite these theoretical objections in practical terms the modified Bernoulli equation has proved to be remarkably accurate in estimating the peak instantaneous pressure difference across the complex lesions of both the right and left ventricular outflow tracts. Continuous wave Doppler is an essential pre-requisite in this respect for both peak velocity estimation and also the evaluation of the respective 'dynamic' and 'fixed' components of the obstruction (Fig. 8 demonstrates the typical waveforms recorded from the right ventricular outflow tract in an infant with Tetralogy of Fallot). The ratio of fixed: dynamic obstruction components may vary among patients with the same anatomic lesion and, in addition, can vary in time in the individual patient. Table 1 demonstrates our findings using continuous wave Doppler to assess the waveforms obtained from 96 children with subvalve stenosis.

Within the left ventricular outflow tract dominant fixed obstructive waveforms were normally found in children with subaortic membranes and fibromuscular tunnels. Dynamic obstruction waveforms were present only in children with hypertropic obstructive cardiomyopathy. Both waveforms were recorded in patients with complex abnormalities of the left ventricular outflow tract. Within the right ventricular outflow tract the common subvalve lesion was part of the spectrum of Tetralogy of Fallot – both fixed and dynamic waveforms were recorded in virtually all these patients. Interestingly, the restriction at the outlet foramen of a univentricular heart could be either a fixed or a dynamic obstruction, with fixed obstruction being the dominant form.

Supravalve stenosis/pulmonary artery banding

Both these entities are fixed obstructive lesions. The gradient across both forms of obstruction is accurately assessed by continuous wave Doppler where either

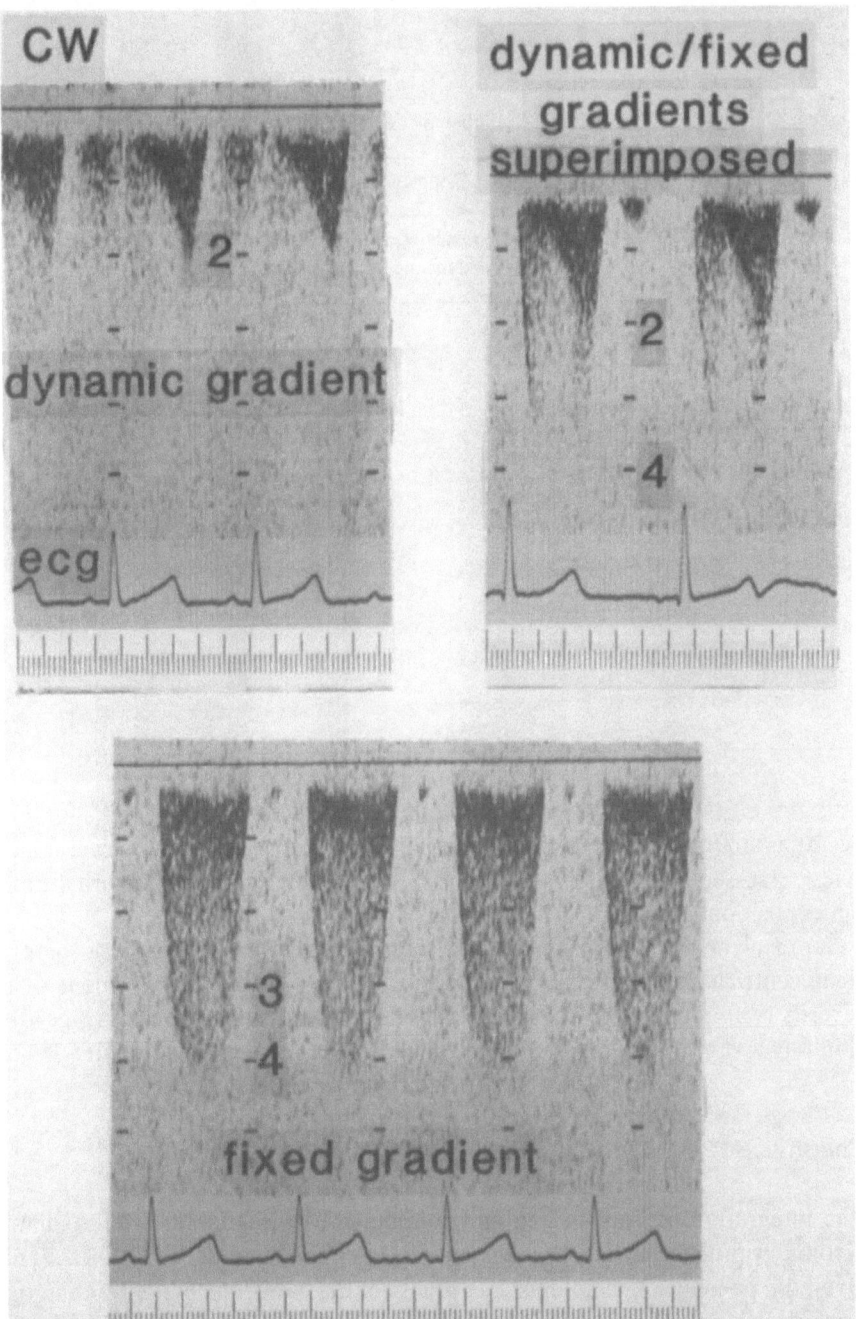

Figure 8. CW Doppler – the characteristic fixed and dynamic obstruction wave-forms recorded from the right ventricular outflow tract in a child with Tetralogy of Fallot.

Upper left panel: With the CW transducer placed in the subcostal position and angulated towards the mid-point of the left clavicle the dynamic obstruction waveform will normally be recorded with no superimposition of the more distal fixed obstruction. Note the characteristic slow increase in the gradient to a late systolic peak of 2 m/second.

Upper right panel: Angulation of the CW transducer towards the mid-line will normally allow both waveforms to be recorded with one superimposed on the other. Note the rapid rise to a peak in early systole of the fixed obstruction gradient.

Lower panel: With more medial and posterior transducer angulation the full waveform of the fixed obstruction will normally be derived in this case reaching a peak gradient equalling 4 m/second.

Table 1. Outflow tract obstruction in CHD Doppler evaluation.

Pts	Lesion	Doppler wave form		
		Isolated dynamic	Isolated fixed	Dynamic and fixed
Isolated obstruction				
13	Sub aortic membrane	–	13	–
5	LV tunnel	–	5	–
11	Restrictive outlet foramen	3	8	–
7	HOCM	7	–	–
4	RVOT infundibular	3	1	–
Multilevel obstruction				
31	Tetralogy of Fallot	–	7	24
9	Complex LVOT obstruction (normal connections)	–	4	5
4	Complex sub-aortic obstruction (univentricular heart)	–	–	4
84				

occurs as an isolated lesion. Isolated supravalvar aortic stenosis is a rare lesion. It is best assessed by interrogating ascending aortic flow from a suprasternal transducer position (Fig. 9).

Supravalvar pulmonary stenosis is virtually always a component of a complex right ventricular outflow tract obstructive lesion. Accurate assessment of its severity is frequently very difficult. Pulmonary artery branch stenosis (Fig. 10) is similarly a very difficult lesion to assess with both imaging and Doppler.

Conclusions

The integration of both pulsed and continuous wave Doppler into paediatric cardiology practice is the major advance in the speciality in the early 1980s. It has given the paediatric cardiologist a certainty of diagnosis much greater than that previously derived from the combination of clinical and cross sectional echo alone. With this certainty of diagnosis of both anatomy and haemodynamics we should see a significant reduction in diagnostic cardiac catheterisation over the next few years. The use of intraoperative duplex scanning will increase significantly allowing the surgeon to assess his repair in theatre. Duplex scanning will become a prerequisite for the study of the natural history of cardiac lesions and for immediate and late post operative assessment. The introduction of colour encoded Doppler should lead to a greater appreciation of abnormal flow patterns

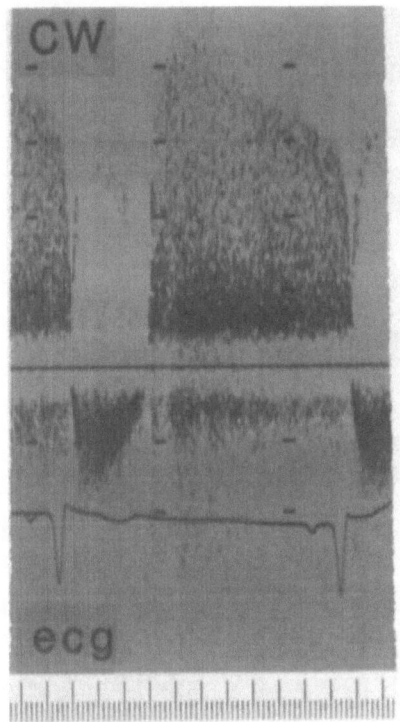 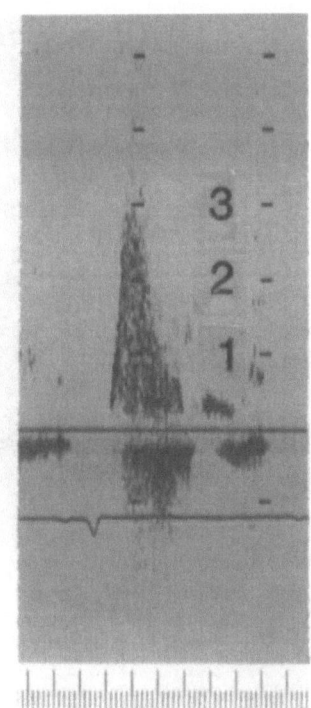

Figure 9. Supra aortic stenosis – a CW Doppler study.

Left hand panel: CW Doppler – apical transducer position. The peak velocity of flow across the left ventricular outflow tract is 1.5 m/second. No gradient exists at aortic valve level. Moderate aortic incompetence is present.

Right hand panel: CW Doppler – suprasternal transducer position. A high velocity jet of 3 m/second was recorded from a suprasternal transducer position. A pulsed Doppler interrogation of the ascending aorta confirmed normal flow velocity above the aortic valve with a subsequent increase in velocity above the coronary sinuses, thus, confirming both the presence and site of the supra aortic stenosis.

and should facilitate the Doppler examination – albeit at considerable financial outlay. However, problem areas still exist. As yet there is no accurate non-invasive method for use in determining pulmonary vascular resistances. Exclusion of the presence of a second VSD in the pre-surgical assessment is impossible. The assessment of atrioventricular and semilunar valve regurgitation remains only a semi-quantitative measurement. More experience is still required to define and circumvent the problem areas in Qp : Qs estimation. All these are potentially soluble problems.

204

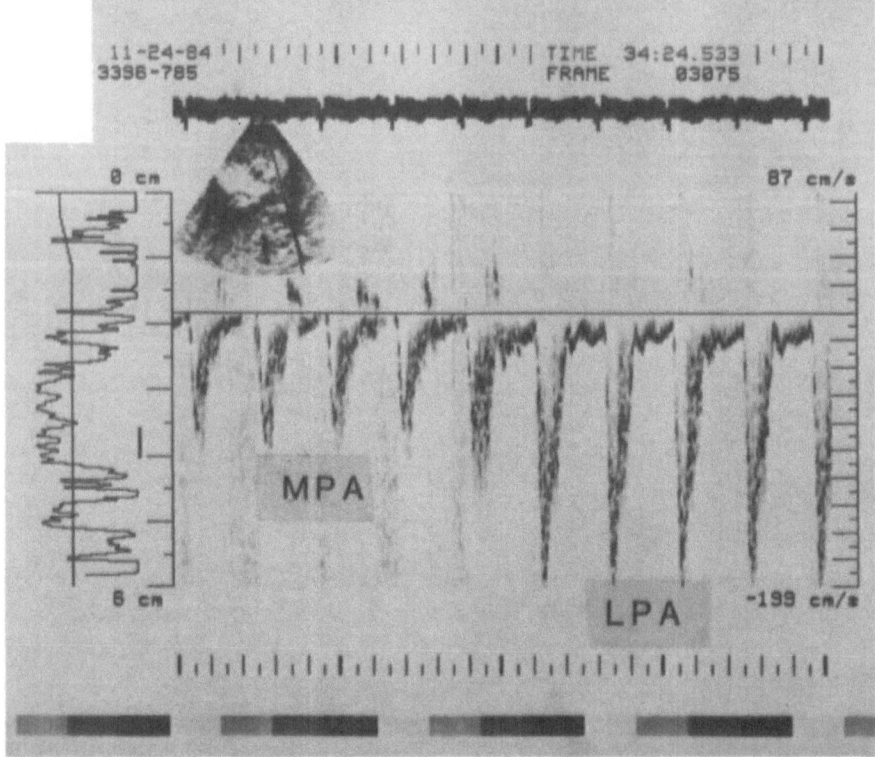

Figure 10. Branch pulmonary artery stenosis – a pulsed Doppler study. In this patient with Tetralogy of Fallot branch pulmonary artery stenosis at the junction of main and left pulmonary artery has been detected by pulsed Doppler. The sample volume has been swept from main to left pulmonary artery and a significant increase in flow velocity has been recorded indicating a stenosis is present. Accurate estimation of the gradient across the branch stenosis is normally impossible in this situation because of the poor alignment of the Doppler beam to flow.

References

1. Stevenson JG, Kawabori I, Dooley T, Guntheroth WG: Diagnosis of ventricular septal defect by pulsed Doppler echocardiography – sensitivity, specificity and limitations. Circulation 58: 322–326, 1978.
2. Hatle L, Rokseth R: Noninvasive diagnosis and assessment of ventricular septal defect by Doppler ultrasound. Acta Med Scand Suppl. 645: 47–56, 1981.
3. Skjaerpe T, Hegrenaes L: Noninvasive estimation of right ventricular pressure by Doppler ultrasound in VSD. In: Fifth Symposium on Echocardiology, Rotterdam 1983. Ultrasonar Bull. 92 (Abstract), 1983.
4. Vargas Barron J, Sahn DJ, Valdes-Cruz LM, Oliveira Lima C, Grenadier E, Allen HD, Goldberg SJ: Quantification of the ration of pulmonary:systemic blood flow (QP : QS) in patients with ventricular septal defect by two-dimensional range gated Doppler echocardiography. Circulation Supp. II: 318 (Abstract), 1982.

5. Stevenson JG, Kawabori I: Sequential 2D echo/Doppler: Improved noninvasive diagnosis of atrial septal defect. Circulation 68 (Suppl III): 110 (Abstract), 1983.

6. Kalmanson D, Veyrat C, Savier CH, Berkman M, Chiche P: Non-invasive technique for diagnosing atrial septal defect and assessing shunt volume using directional Doppler ultrasound. Br Heart J 34: 981–991, 1972.

7. Colvin EV, Gutgesell HP, Cohen M, Bricker T, Latson LA: Assessment of pulmonary to systemic flow ratio in normal children by Doppler and two-dimensional echocardiography. J Am Coll Cardiol 1: 682 (Abstract), 1983.

8. Stevenson JG, Kawabori I: Noninvasive determination of pulmonic to systemic flow ratio by pulsed Doppler echo. Circulation 66 (Suppl. II): 232 (Abstract), 1982.

9. Fischer DC, Sahn DJ, Friedman MJ, Larson D, Valdes-Cruz LM, Horowitz S, Goldberg SJ, Allen HD: The mitral valve orifice method for non-invasive two-dimensional echo Doppler determination of cardiac output. Circulation 67: 872–877, 1983.

10. Stevenson JG, Kawabori I, Guntheroth WG: Pulsed Doppler echocardiographic diagnosis of patent ductus arteriosus: sensitivity, specificity, limitations and technical features. Cathet Cardiovasc Diagn 6: 255–263, 1980.

11. Stevenson JG, Dooley TK, Kawabori I: Patent ductus arteriosus in a neonatal intensive care unit: the utility of pulsed Doppler echocardiography. Circulation 58 (Suppl. III): 110 (Abstract), 1978.

12. Serwer GA, Armstrong BE, Anderson PAW: Continuous wave Doppler ultrasonographic quantitation of patent ductus arteriosus flow. J Paediatr 100: 297–329, 1982.

Assessment of the clinical value of continuous wave Doppler ultrasound in children with acyanotic congenital heart disease

A.B. Houston, I.A. Simpson and C.D. Sheldon

Introduction

Echocardiography, particularly the cross-sectional technique, now provides so accurate a demonstration of intracardiac anatomy that surgery in congenital defects can often be undertaken without angiocardiography. However in acyanotic lesions indications for surgery are often based not simply on the presence of the lesion but rather its haemodynamic effects such as the severity of obstruction, the pulmonary artery pressure or resistance, or the magnitude of an intracardiac shunt. Some information on this can be obtained from M-mode echocardiography by assessing the chamber sizes, wall thickness and valve motion but more detailed information is frequently required making cardiac catheterisation mandatory in assessing the need for surgery.

Although Doppler ultrasound has been used in cardiology for a considerable time, wide interest in its value in congenital heart disease has only developed in the last few years, largely due to the efforts of Hatle and her colleagues [1] using both pulsed and continuous wave Doppler. The use of continuous wave Doppler, with the application of the Bernoulli formula, is potentially of great value in congenital defects where measurement of pressure gradients or absolute pressures is usually more important than calculations of flow. Findings in a wide variety of congenital defects have been described by Hatle et al. and other groups and we have applied this technique in a consecutive series of patients admitted for catheterisation of surgery. This report will describe mainly those with acyanotic congenital heart disease in whom a gradient might be expected who were undergoing cardiac catheterisation (75), admitted for surgery having previously been catheterised (21), or undergoing surgery without catheterisation (10). To provide sufficient numbers with infundibular stenosis for statistical analysis 12 children with Tetralogy of Fallot were included whether they were cyanosed or not. It includes only those in whom a gradient was demonstrated or might be expected to be found, namely pulmonary stenosis at valve (26) or infundibular (23) level, pulmonary artery band (3), aortic stenosis (12), coarctation complex (21) and VSD (21).

Cardiac catheterisation was performed under sedation, the pressures on either side of the lesion being measured using a fluid filled catheter attached to a Statham transducer. The gradient across the obstructive lesion was obtained as a peak-to-peak pressure difference, where possible from a withdrawal tracing. In some patients variations in pressure with respiration or the occurrence of ectopic beats on catheter withdrawal made exact measurement of pressures difficult; in these cases tracings were reviewed by an independent observer who, by averaging the cycles, decided on an appropriate systolic pressure.

The ultrasound equipment consisted of an ATL sector scanner and a separate multifrequency continuous and pulsed wave Doppler unit (Alfred, Vingmed) which was used in the continuous mode with a 2 MHz transducer. The Doppler shifted audio signal was monitored on a spectrum analyser (Angioscan or Doptek) fitted with a movable marker line which aided judgement of the level of the received Doppler shift in relation to the preceeding investigation.

A two-dimensional echocardiogram was first obtained to demonstrate the intracardiac anatomy and suggest the position from which the ultrasound beam might best be aligned parallel to flow through the obstructive lesion. The Doppler study was then performed to obtain the optimum Doppler signal showing the highest frequency shift by setting the gain on the spectrum analyser to give the maximum signal without obvious noise and making appropriate adjustments to the position and angulation of the probe. As different positions were explored the marker line on the spectrum analyser was moved, as necessary, to the level of the average of the received maximum Doppler signals ignoring occasional ones of higher frequency. At the end of the examination the level (in KHz) of the line on the spectrum analyser giving maximum Doppler frequency shift was noted (Fig. 1), the velocity in metres per second calculated, and the pressure drop obtained from the modified Bernoulli formula, $P = 4V^2$, where P = pressure gradient (mmHg) and V = maximum velocity (m/sec) [2].

Pulmonary valve stenosis or arterial band

Twenty-nine children (aged 5 weeks to 15 years, mean 5.3 years) were studied. All underwent cardiac catheterisation because of suspected pulmonary stenosis (24) or for reassessment following pulmonary valvotomy (2) or pulmonary artery banding (3). One had combined pulmonary valve and branch stenosis, six an associated ventricular septal defect, one an atrial septal defect, and one an absent pulmonary valve with significant stenosis and regurgitation.

Nineteen patients underwent the Doppler study while sedated for cardiac catheterisation, the study being performed as the catheter was withdrawn across the obstruction in 7, immediately after withdrawal in 7, and while simultaneous pulmonary arterial and right ventricular pressures were measured in 5. In the patients studied at catheterisation the peak-to-peak pressure gradients ranged

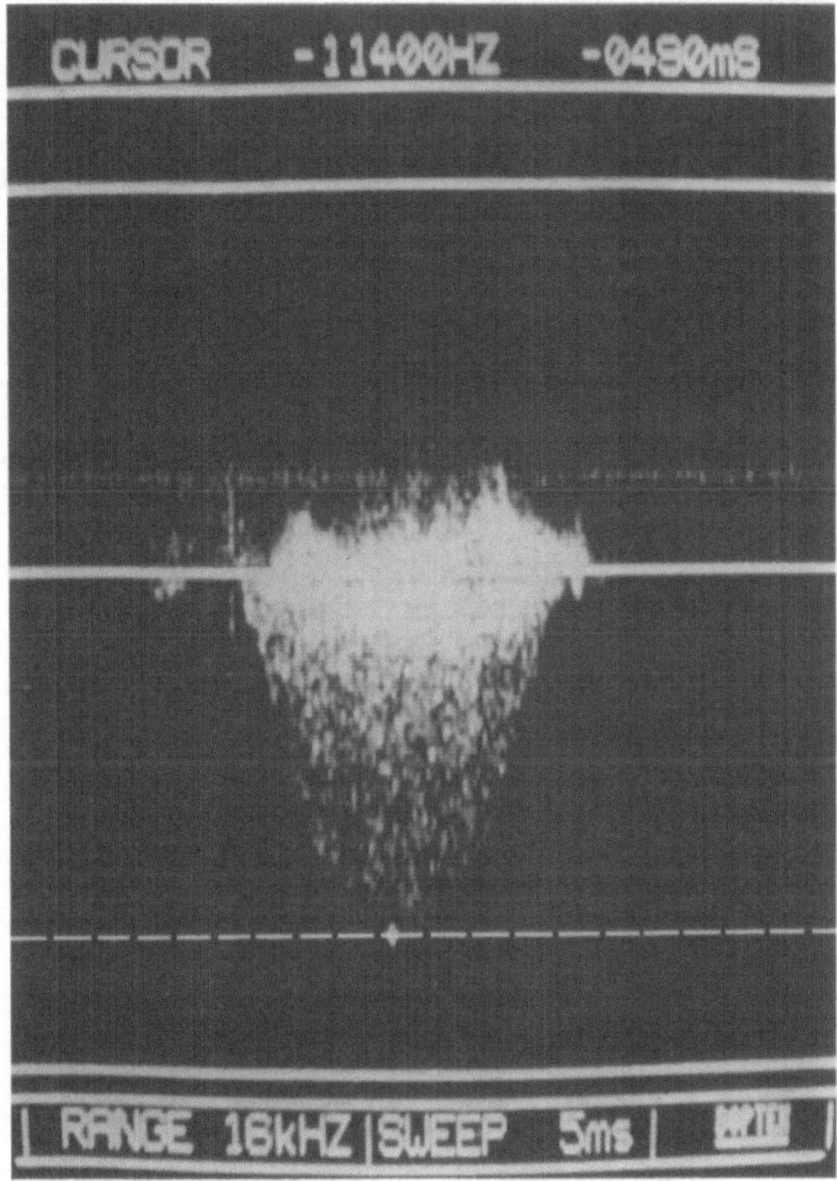

Figure 1. Recording of the Doppler signal from the spectrum analyser from a patient with pulmonary valve stenosis. The signal is negative indicating flow away from the transducer. The maximum frequency shift of 11,400 Hz (indicated by the dotted marker line) represents a velocity of 4.5 m/sec and a gradient of 79 mmHg.

from 10–226 mmHg by manometry and from 15–189 mmHg from Doppler calculation. In the 7 patients in whom the Doppler signal was recorded during catheter withdrawal no change in the maximum velocity occurred during this procedure. Comparison of the gradients is shown in Fig. 2. The regression analysis excludes the patient with a measured gradient of 226 mmHg (189 mmHg by Doppler) since her inclusion would have reduced the slope of the regression line, although the correlation co-efficient would have been increased. This exclusion was considered appropriate since such high gradients are unusual in pulmonary stenosis, and it is known that Doppler will underestimate the gradient across a very narrow orifice [3] because Bernoulli's equation does not take into account losses due to viscous effects. Several studies [1, 4, 5] including our own [6] attest to the accuracy of continuous wave Doppler in the measurement of pressure gradient in pulmonary valve stenosis. Other workers have tended to show that this will not be overestimated whereas this has occurred in some of our patients. This may be due to changes in the gradient in non simultaneous studies or the use of the moving

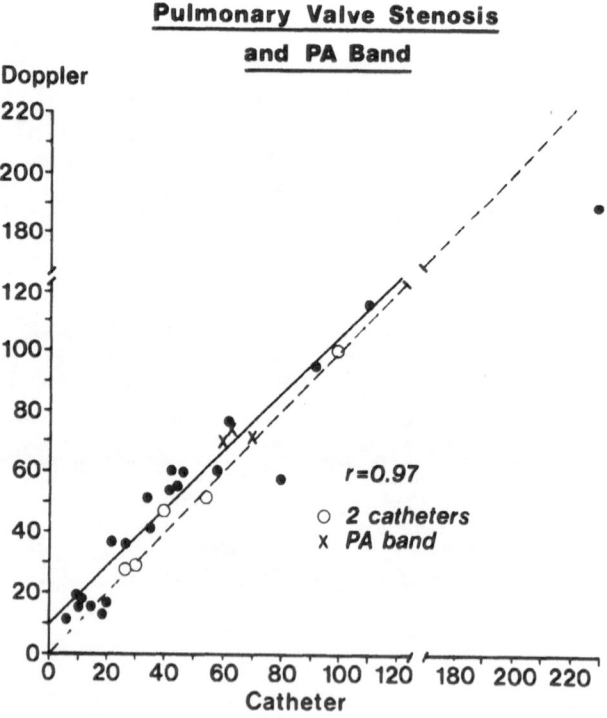

Figure 2. Comparison of the pressure gradients measured at catheterisation and estimated with Doppler in the 29 patients with pulmonary valve stenosis. As explained in the text the patient with a measured gradient of 226 mmHg is excluded from the linear regression line which has a gradient of 0.94 (y = 0.94x + 9.8). Abbreviations: 0 = pressure measured with 2 catheters; x = pulmonary artery band.

line on the spectrum analyser to ensure that the highest average set of recordings is taken. However study of the 5 patients in whom the gradient was recorded simultaneously with pressure measurement using two catheters has shown a very close correlation with the recorded values (Fig. 2) and since these should be the most accurate measurements this suggests that the Doppler technique is sufficiently accurate for clinical purposes.

Pulmonary infundibular stenosis

Twenty-three infants and children (7 days to 16 years, mean 2.8 years) with infundibular pulmonary stenosis were studied by cardiac catheterisation, although it was not possible to enter the pulmonary artery in 6. Eleven had infundibular and possible valve stenosis (9 with a VSD) and 12 tetralogy of Fallot. The gradient was measured from pressures obtained as the catheter was advanced from the right ventricle to the pulmonary artery. In 15 the Doppler study was performed with the child sedated at the time of catheterisation and in the other 8 at the time of admission for subsequent surgery. The Doppler study was not performed during catheter withdrawal because of possible complications related to infundibular obstruction.

Satisfactory Doppler recordings were obtained from all patients. Maximum blood flow velocities were obtained almost equally frequently from subxyphoid and parasternal positions. Comparison of the maximum Doppler gradient with the measured one showed a correlation coefficient of 0.94 with $y = 0.92x + 6.97$.

Several studies attest to the accuracy of Doppler ultrasound in measuring the gradient in infants and children with discrete pulmonary valve stenosis [1, 4, 5, 6] but there is little information on infundibular stenosis [1, 5]. The formula as described by Bernoulli relates the pressure gradient to the kinetic energy content of a fluid before and after an obstruction, and this will not change whether the obstruction is discrete or elongated. However the application of the modified formula $P = 4V^2$ assumes there is no energy loss due to friction, which may become more important the longer the length of the obstruction or where it occurs at more than one level, as can happen in infundibular stenosis. However the results of this study are in accord with those previously reported with discrete obstruction and indicate that the modified Bernoulli formula can be applied in infundibular pulmonary stenosis.

Aortic stenosis

Twelve patients with aortic stenosis were studied, including some with subvalve and supravalve obstruction. Catheterisation was performed in 10 but in 3 the left ventricle could not be entered through the aortic valve and direct puncture was

212

considered unnecessary in view of the Doppler findings. Comparison of the gradients showed a satisfactory correlation (Fig. 3) although the numbers are rather small for statistical analysis. The patient in whom the gradient was markedly underestimated had subvalve, valve,and supravalve stenosis with a very distorted outflow tract, making it impossible for the Doppler beam to be aligned along the length of the obstructed region. However Doppler correctly predicted that the obstructive lesion was of significance while echocardiography showed the very abnormal outflow. Thus if the two techniques are taken together a reliable assessment of the severity of aortic stenosis should be obtained.

Ventricular septal defect

Twenty-one infants and children (aged 5 weeks to 8 years) were studied, 18 when sedated for catheterisation. At catheterisation the left and right ventricular pressures were measured using a single catheter and were thus not simultaneous. The Doppler study was performed as close as possible to the time when these

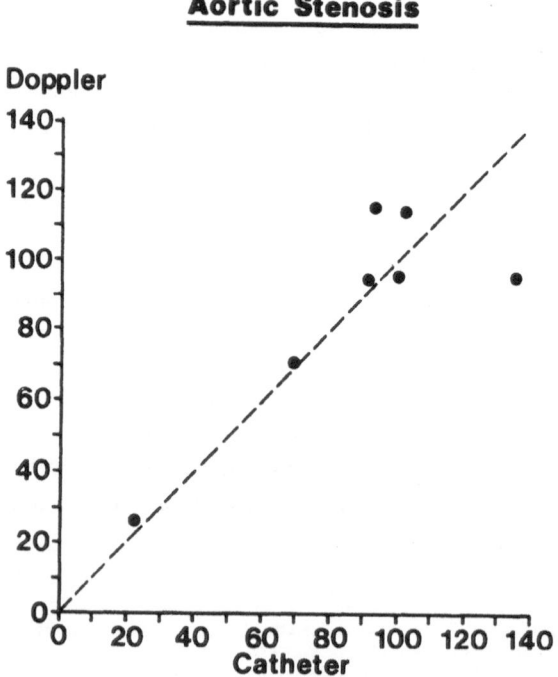

Figure 3. Comparison of pressure gradients measured at catheterisation and estimated with Doppler in the 7 patients with aortic stenosis in whom it was possible to measure the left ventricular pressure at catheterisation. Statistical analysis has not been performed because of the small numbers.

measurements were made, the maximum velocity being measured only after exploring a wide variety of sites. When no VSD jet could be located the decision that there was no ventricular pressure difference (and thus systemic level right ventricular pressure) was made only after every effort had been made from all possible praecordial and subxyphoid positions. In all cases the Doppler shift was positive indicating flow towards the transducer. It was occasionally difficult to obtain a spectral signal with a clear cut peak and then the maximum part of the spectral signal was measured with the knowledge that this might be less than the true maximum.

Comparison of the pressure difference at catheterisation (0 to 108 mmHg) and from Doppler (0 to 98 mmHg) is shown in Figure 4. In 2 patients the pressure gradient was considerably underestimated and the regression line falls below the line of identity which, in comparison to the findings in pulmonary valve stenosis, suggests a tendency for Doppler to underestimate the true difference; this may be because of problems in aligning along the jet because of movement of the ventricular septum with cardiac contraction.

The results, however, are similar to those of Hatle et al. [1] and demonstrate the validity of using Doppler ultrasound to assess the systolic pressure difference

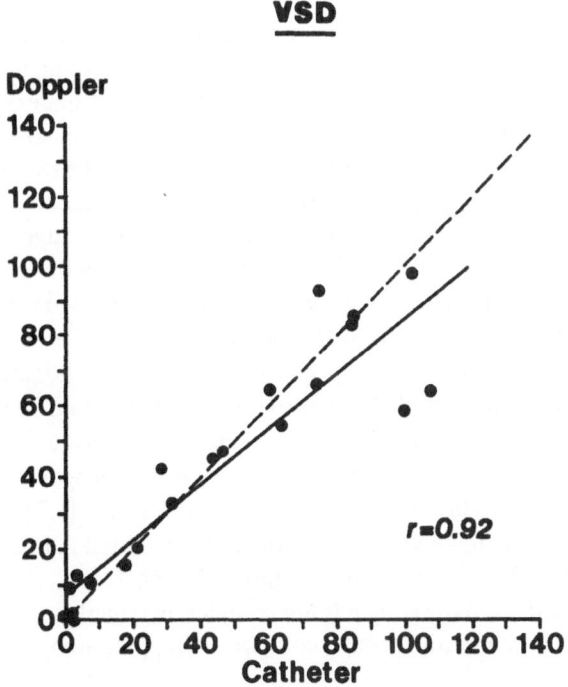

Figure 4. Comparison of pressure gradients measured at catheterisation and estimated with Doppler in 21 patients with a VSD (y = 0.79x + 8.3).

between the ventricles. Since the left ventricular systolic pressure equals that of the systolic blood pressure which can be measured with a sphygmomanometer or electronic system the right ventricular systolic pressure can be calculated. Providing there is no pulmonary stenosis (confirmed by Doppler) this will equal the pulmonary artery systolic pressure. The major potential error is underestimation of the pressure gradient due to failure to align the ultrasound beam in the direction of flow, but since this will result in an overestimation of the right ventricle and pulmonary artery pressures those with pulmonary hypertension will not be missed.

Coarctation complex

Twenty-one patients (13 infants and 8 older children) were studied. The diagnosis of coarctation of the aorta was established by catheterisation in 11, and by echocardiography and subsequent surgery in 8. The two remaining patients had an interrupted aortic arch with a patent ductus arteriosus.

Doppler recordings were made from the suprasternal notch the transducer being first angled to show flow up the ascending aorta (positive frequency shift) and then tilted to show flow in the region of the arch and proximal descending aorta (negative shift). In 18 of the 19 patients with coarctation this demonstrated an increase in blood flow velocity from the ascending to the descending aorta (Fig. 5) indicating a pressure drop across the coarctation. No high velocity in the aortic arch could be demonstrated in one child who had undergone repair of coarctation of the aorta when only 1.2 kg; subsequent surgery showed her to have a long segment narrowing with a very narrow diameter. In the two infants with an interrupted aortic arch a high velocity negative signal was obtained with the transducer angled to the distal arch and descending aorta suggesting the possibility of coarctation. It is likely that this flow was through the ductus from the pulmonary artery to the descending aorta and the use of pulsed wave Doppler to attempt to follow aortic flow from the proximal arch to the descending aorta might have obviated the error. Similarly it is possible that in the case where no jet was recorded the use of pulsed Doppler to map the flow would demonstrate that there was no flow from the distal arch to the descending aorta.

These results are similar to previous reports on the recognition of gradients across a coarctation as a high velocity jet from the distal arch [1, 7]. However they indicate that a jet may not always be demonstrated and that in infants ductal fow may be mistaken for the coarctation. Thus although Doppler ultrasound can usually demonstrate a coarctation it is not completely reliable and false negatives and false positives can occur if continuous wave Doppler alone is used.

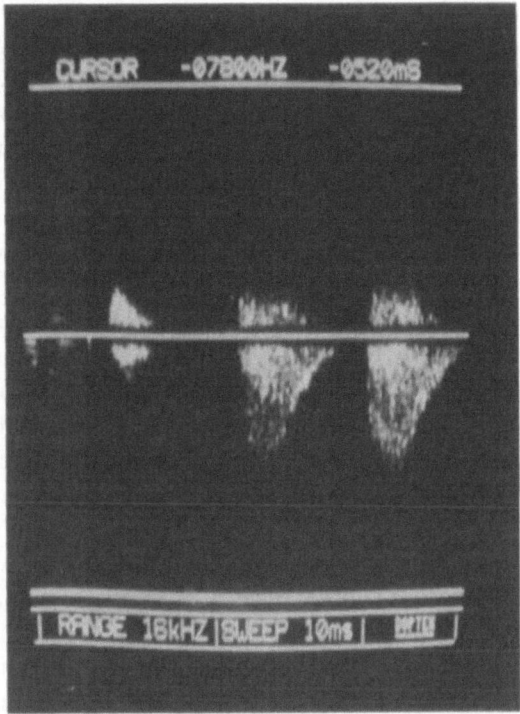

Figure 5. Recording of the Doppler signal from the spectrum analyser from a patient with coarctation of the aorta. The transducer is placed in the suprasternal notch and tilted from the ascending to descending aorta. Flow in the ascending aorta is towards the transducer (positive) while that in the distal arch is away from it (negative) and of higher velocity.

Discussion

The results of this study are in keeping with the work of others demonstrating the application of the Bernoulli formula to provide an accurate assessment of pressure drop. There are of course potential errors, particularly related to difficulties in aligning the ultrasound beam along the jet when no attempt is made to correct for the angle of incidence. It has therefore become appropriate to consider the place that, in the future, continuous wave Doppler may adopt in the management of the more common and less common complex types of congenital heart disease. In this study two common acyanotic lesions, patent ductus arteriosus (PDA) and atrial septal defect (ASD), have not been considered. In our practice patients with PDA or ASD generally undergo surgery without catheterisation, and it has not been possible to obtain comparative information between catheterisation and Doppler in these conditions. The ability of Doppler to demonstrate flow reversal in the distal aortic arch of flow into the pulmonary artery in PDA may prove to be valuable in the premature infant or the more complex lesion with a PDA, but although it will provide confirmatory evidence of the diagnosis it is unlikely to prove essential in the assessment of the majority of patients with this lesion. The diagnosis of a secundum ASD and the need for surgery is usually readily apparent with clinical examination and echocardiographic demonstration of a large right ventricle, paradoxical septal motion, and a hole in the atrial septum. Pulsed wave Doppler can estimate the shunt size non-invasively but it is time consuming and in most cases is unnecessary in deciding whether catheterisation or surgery is necessary. However it is prudent to use Doppler to ensure there is no significant pulmonary stenosis or tricuspid regurgitation.

The site and size of a significant VSD can usually be demonstrated by cross-sectional echocardiography and although shunt size is useful, knowledge of pulmonary artery pressure is more important. In the infant with a VSD who is failing to thrive or in whom cardiac failure cannot be controlled medically the need for surgery is readily apparent, while in the asymptomatic child VSD closure will be necessary before two years old if there is pulmonary hypertension. Although this can be suspected on clinical grounds or from non-invasive tests such as the ECG, or right ventricular systolic time intervals on M-mode echocardiography, none of these is entirely reliable. A variety of methods for assessing pulmonary artery pressure with Doppler have been reported, continuous wave lending itself particularly to the measurement of right ventricular (and thus pulmonary arterial) pressure by picking up a jet of tricuspid regurgition (right ventricular to right atrial pressure difference) or through the VSD (left to right ventricular difference). A possible error with these may occur with underestimation of the pressure drop due to failure to pick up the jet or to obtain a small enough angle to the line of flow. With the former technique there is a theoretical danger of underestimating the right ventricular pressure. However if the VSD jet is used underestimation of the pressure drop will overestimate the right ventricular (and pulmonary arterial) pressure and those with a high pulmonary artery pressure will not be missed although some may be incorrectly thought to have pulmonary hypertension. If the technique is used to select those with a VSD who require catheterisation, all patients needing surgery should be included. Where a jet cannot be recorded through the VSD other techniques such as the measurement of the tricuspid regurgitant jet [1] may prove useful.

In pulmonary valve stenosis surgery is considered necessary where the gradient across the valve is 40–50 mmHg. Significant obstruction can be suspected where there is evidence of right ventricular hypertrophy on clinical or ECG examination or a widely split second sound with a soft pulmonary component, but echocardiography is of little help. The accuracy of Doppler ultrasound in measuring pulmonary gradients suggests the results are sufficiently reliable to base clinical decisions on it. Thus a Doppler gradient of less than 30 mmHg would mean the obstruction is not significant whereas one greater than 50 mmHg would mean that surgery or angioplasty was required. A value between 30 and 50 might be surgically significant but the obstruction will not be severe and it may be appropriate to defer surgery or angioplasty and perform serial Doppler studies. Since the Bernoulli formula appears to hold for patients with infundibular stenosis Doppler should also assist in the management of these patients and it has been able to assess the pressure gradient in patients where this could not be measured because of the potential hazard of passing a catheter through a severely narrowed outflow tract. In many of these patients Doppler may be superfluous since clinical and echocardiographic assessment will indicate the need for angiocardiography or surgical treatment. However there are others in whom the degree of infundibular stenosis may alter with time and serial Doppler measurement will be useful in follow up.

Although the numbers with aortic stenosis are small the results are in agreement with those of previous studies in children [1, 8] showing the technique to be as valid as in pulmonary stenosis. This will assist with decisions as to whether full exercise will be permissible, exercise should be limited, or investigation and possible surgery are required.

In most cases of coarctation of the aorta the diagnosis is made clinically and its site can be demonstrated with echocardiography. There are however some patients from whom clear echocardiographic images cannot be obtained and another non-invasive technique to confirm the site would be useful. However the results described here suggest that although Doppler ultrasound can usually demonstrate a coarctation it is not completely reliable and false negatives and false positives can occur if continuous wave Doppler alone is used. Particular care must be exercised in the newborn with a right to left shunt through a PDA, where ductal flow can be mistaken for that through a coarctation.

In applying Doppler ultrasound to the conditions discussed here continuous wave Doppler has been essential to measure high velocities. It has the additional advantage over pulsed Doppler in that the study is easier and therefore takes less time. However even for a continuous wave Doppler study the patient must be co-operative and lie still for sufficiently long to allow a full examination to be performed. Most of the patients described here were examined when sedated for catheterisation; in some an attempt to examine them before this proved impossible because of poor co-operation. Thus practical application of Doppler ultrasound in the older infant and toddler may require sedation. However, the results provide information of such clinical value that this will be justified and, in some cases, preclude the need for catheterisation.

At present it seems the results are accurate and provide important and reliable information in those with semi-lunar valve stenosis, including infundibular stenosis and pulmonary artery banding, whereas in VSD and coarctation the findings can often be useful, but should for the meantime be interpreted with caution. It is likely in the future that the place of continuous wave Doppler will be confirmed and strengthened and, as part of the whole non-invasive examination, further improve the care of the infant and child with congenital heart disease.

References

1. Hatle L, Angelsen B: Doppler Ultrasound in Cardiology. Physical principles and clinical applications (2nd ed.). Philadelphia: Lea and Febiger, 1985.
2. Hatle L, Brubakk A, Tromsdal A, Angelsen B: Non-invasive assessment of pressure drop in mitral stenosis by Doppler ultrasound. Br Heart J 40: 131–40, 1978.
3. Holen J, Aaslid R, Landmark K, Simonsen S, Ostrem T: Determination of effective orifice area in mitral stenosis from non-invasive ultrasound Doppler data and mitral flow rate. Acta Med Scand 201: 83–8, 1977.
4. Lima CO, Sahn DJ, Valdes-Cruz LM, *et al.*: Non-invasive prediction of transvalvular pressure gradient in patients with pulmonary stenosis by quantitative two-dimensional echocardiographic Doppler studies. Circulation 67: 866–71, 1983.
5. Johnson GL, Kwan OL, Handshoe S, Noonan JA, DE Maria AN: Accuracy of combined two-dimensional echocardiography and continuous wave Doppler recordings in the estimation of pressure gradient in right ventricular outlet obstruction. JACC 3: 1013–8, 1984.
6. Houston AB, Sheldon CS, Simpson IA, Doig WB, Coleman EN: The severity of pulmonary valve or artery obstruction in children estimated by Doppler ultrasound. Eur Heart J 1985; in press.
7. Wyse RK, Robinson PJ, Deanfield JE, Tunstall Pedoe DS, Macartney FJ: Use of continuous wave Doppler ultrasound velocimetry to assess the severity of coarctation of the aorta by measurement of aortic flow velocities. Br Heart J 52: 278–83, 1984.
8. Lima CO, Sahn DJ, Valdes-Cruz LM, *et al.*: Prediction of the severity of left ventricular outlet obstruction by quantitative two-dimensional echocardiographic Doppler studies. Circulation 68: 348–54, 1983.

Index